WASHED
in the BLOOD

a true story about TRIUMPH
over remarkable circumstances

JERRY WILDE

NEW YORK

WASHED *in the* BLOOD
a true story about TRIUMPH *over remarkable circumstances*

by JERRY WILDE

ISBN 978-1-61448-052-5 (paperback)
ISBN 978-1-61448-053-2 (eBook)

Published by:
MORGAN JAMES PUBLISHING
The Entrepreneurial Publisher
5 Penn Plaza, 23rd Floor
New York City, New York 10001
(212) 655-5470 Office
(516) 908-4496 Fax
www.MorganJamesPublishing.com

Cover Design by:
Rachel Lopez
rachel@r2cdesign.com

Interior Design by:
Bonnie Bushman
bbushman@bresnan.net

Photo Credits:
Indiana University East
Susanna Tanner

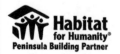

In an effort to support local communities, raise awareness and funds, Morgan James Publishing donates one percent of all book sales for the life of each book to Habitat for Humanity.
Get involved today, visit
www.HelpHabitatForHumanity.org.

ACKNOWLEDGEMENTS

To my wife - thank you for being my candle when all I could see was darkness.

To my children - I love you more than words can say. I am sorry my illness has taken away from your carefree childhoods. Perhaps you have learned some lessons about handling adversity.

To the nurses and techs at the Fresenius Dialysis Center in Richmond, Indiana - thank you for keeping me alive long enough to write this book. To the nocturnal crew (Lori, Heather, and Trey), much love and respect. You make the unbearable, bearable.

To the people who have volunteered to be tested to be donors - thank you for giving me hope. Because of you, I have never felt alone on this journey.

IT HAD TO BE THE PIZZA GUY

It was a Thursday afternoon. The day had been long and, as I recall, not exactly a good one. An early morning meeting after teaching an evening class the night before had me yawning before lunch. The afternoon was spent in a long meeting with my colleagues from the School of Education. These meetings are not fun or sexy. The phrase "necessary evil" springs to mind as we trudged through the minutia of our programs. Everyone in the room recognized that we have to meet to take care of business, but after a dozen years of these weekly meetings, let's just say the "thrill was gone." I was looking forward to getting home if for no other reason than it was a change of scenery from the office. However, my usual routine carried no clue of what was to come.

They say that you never really recognize the important moments of your life while they are happening. Who are "they?" I'm not exactly sure but I know I've heard that before. It seems like it was a Woody Allen movie. Well, regardless of who said it, I beg to differ. There are certain cases when you have a clear recognition that the moment you are experiencing will change your life forever. That was certainly the case on that day in October of 2009. I was just ready to head home when the phone rang. It was a call from the nurse practitioner I had seen earlier in the week. For the past couple of weeks I had been experiencing flu-like symptoms. A low-grade fever, nausea, and weakness were the most prevalent symptoms but there were a couple of others that seemed odd. My skin itched and my urine was very dark. This "flu" wiped me out for a couple of days so the change in the color of my urine, I assumed, was related to slight dehydration.

About a week later I came down with identical symptoms. Now, I am not a doctor (not the medical kind anyway) but I knew that having a viral infection would make it highly unlikely that I would get the same flu a week later. My wife had been worried about me as I think she sensed that perhaps this wasn't just a case of the flu. Polly had been searching through the physician's desk reference, which she loves to do, and came up with my diagnosis. "I think you might have hepatitis," proclaimed Mrs. Dr. Wilde.

Like all good husbands, I hated the idea of my wife being correct about anything, especially about something important. "I don't have hepatitis. I wish you'd put that damn thing away," I protested.

"Oh yeah? Come here and look at these symptoms," she said. After looking over the symptoms, I had to admit that her diagnostic skills were impressive. Everything on the list, I had! "Shit. How the heck did I get hepatitis?" I had recently taken a trip to Washington D.C. for a conference and I immediately started to click off the list of possible hepatitis carriers in my head. It could have been the guy driving the van to the hotel but I doubt it. He seemed fine. Maybe it was the check-in lady but that seems doubtful. Then it dawned on me. It had to be the pizza guy! He looked a little funky and he had handled my food. Damn! I was felled by my love of pizza. Somehow it seemed appropriate. It was almost like this plot came out of a modern day Shakespearian tragedy.

Even though my wife had worked her diagnostic magic with the PDR I thought it would be prudent to consult with a real doctor to confirm her diagnosis. I assured her she would get full credit for the "catch" which seemed to please her. I set up an appointment with my doctor but he was busy so I thought it would be best to see the first practitioner available. After all, my wife had this thing nailed. How hard was it to order a blood test? I ended up seeing a nurse practitioner a couple of days later. She poked and prodded me and afterwards said, "Well your liver doesn't seem enlarged but I'd like you to have an ultrasound just to make sure." I left the office that day without having a blood test for hepatitis. "Typical," I thought. "Damn doctors always ordering tests just to soak some money out of my insurance company. They can't stand it when the patients already know what's wrong with them." I reluctantly agreed to have the ultrasound at our local hospital a few days later.

On the day of my ultrasound I was secretly dreading the moment when they put the lubricating goo on me because it's always freezing cold which causes my testicles to disappear into my abdominal cavity and reside somewhere in the general vicinity of my pancreas. It had been years since I had an ultrasound and I was thrilled to learn some kind soul had invented a goo-warming machine. Give that person a Noble Prize immediately! I was on the table as happy as a pig in slop as they rubbed the probe all over my belly. The tech kept going over a certain area of my abdomen again and again.

I finally asked, "Are you looking for something?"

She said, "Your kidneys. I can't seem to find them."

I told her, "I have something called Alport syndrome which made my kidneys stop working years ago. I wouldn't be surprised if my kidneys were just shriveled up and gone."

She made a few more passes before giving up and continuing with the procedure. When she got to the location of my transplanted kidney, she took several pictures and used the function on the machine that uses dotted lines to map the size and location of an object. This didn't surprise me. Who wouldn't be interested in my transplanted kidney? That kidney was a hero. Seventeen years baby! Seventeen years and not a hint of trouble; no rejections, no infections…nothing. This kidney was a certified pee-making machine. In several Latin American countries the natives sing folk songs about Jerry Wilde's transplanted kidney. The tech wiped the somewhat cooler goo off me and I went to teach my class feeling slightly sticky.

A few days later, after a long day of meetings, I was ready to head home when the phone rang in my office. It was the nurse practitioner calling with my results. "Mr. Wilde, I wanted to let you know that your liver shows no signs of being enlarged. That is what I expected to find but now we know for certain."

"I guess it's better to be safe than sorry," I offered getting ready to ask why they were refusing to do a blood test for hepatitis. Before I had the chance to ask the nurse practitioner uttered the words that no one wants to hear.

"There was a rather large mass on your kidney." When people hear words like that there is an initial sense of shock. Did I hear that correctly? A mass on my kidney. What does that mean? Didn't she know about my kidney? Maybe we could just tell the heroic kidney about the mass and Sidney the kidney could kick its ass? But somehow my old friend denial had taken the afternoon off just when I needed him most. I would suspect many people do all sorts of mental gymnastics to cope with the anxiety brought about by the thought of a tumor growing in their body. But sitting there in my office, I could not avoid the thought that my life was going to change forever as a result of this news and this change would not be good.

SO NOW WHAT?

I was reeling from the news that I had a tumor on my transplanted kidney. How? What? Are you sure? Is it big? There were so many questions and no answers. But one of the things I learned years ago when I became sick was that your life does not stop. You keep on living. I remember thinking as a kid, "How do people who have cancer just go about their day? How do they buy groceries and watch TV like nothing is wrong?" I understand now. They do it because they don't have a choice.

I gathered my things and headed home. Once home I checked in with my kids to see how their days had been. It was a beautiful fall day so I said to my wife, "How about taking the dogs for a walk?" We liked walking our dogs and in late October it's wise to enjoy as many nice afternoons as possible with winter just around the corner. We made it about halfway out of our driveway before I said, "We need to talk." Instantly Polly knew something was very, very wrong. I had used that phrase exactly one other time. It was many years ago when I had to tell her I had something called Alport Syndrome and that soon my kidneys would completely shut down. There was no mistaking what that phrase meant to us. It had a history. And I pray to God I never utter those words again.

As expected, our conversation was punctuated with many questions.

"How big is this mass?" she asked.

"They said it was 11 cm," I answered.

"How big is that?" Polly asked.

"I guess it's about the size of a large orange," I replied wondering how it was possible to have a mass the size of a large orange in my belly and not realize it. Many more questions followed. It wasn't until she mentioned our children that she cried. At some point, Theo, our oldest dog, took a massive dump.

My brother Jim is a doctor so it seemed like an excellent time to give him a call. He also had a bunch of questions. As would be expected, he wanted to get a copy of the ultrasound report, which I did not have. He explained that it is not uncommon for a growth like this to be a large cyst filled with fluid. If that were the case, this ominous sounding mass would not result in any serious health problems. It would have to be removed but the thought of surgery is not horrifying; not when you've been through the things I've experienced. A little more abdominal surgery wouldn't be a big deal. My belly already looked like a road map of scars from surgeries for an appendectomy, a kidney transplant, and the insertion and removal of a catheter for peritoneal dialysis. I was much relieved and told my wife that this may be no big deal. This was the start of several emotional roller coasters we would ride over the coming months.

I got a copy of the ultrasound report, which was difficult to understand but one sentence did stand out. The report mentioned "a solid mass highly suspicious of renal cell carcinoma." So…shit. I faxed the report to my brother and waited to hear from him. He emailed a couple of hours later and explained that a solid mass was not good news but that there was still much to be done. He said that an ultrasound is not a very precise instrument and that the doctors would probably want either a MRI or CT scan. No need to panic. There would be plenty of time for panic later.

THE WAITING IS THE HARDEST PART

A week later I found myself being sucked into the giant metallic cylinder of an MRI machine. I was told that it was important to get a more precise scan of this thing but I think the real issue was trying to determine if there were other tumors in the surrounding organs. Of course, if this mass had spread it would be a very bad sign. I wasn't really worried about the findings. As strange as this may sound, I was almost too numb to be worried.

One interesting thing about the MRI machine at our local hospital is that this model actually allowed me to watch TV while a huge magnet was spinning around me. The technicians were very proud of this new MRI machine and I must say it was nice being able to watch a live basketball game during the procedure. It happened to be a special day for college basketball. ESPN was running some sort of promotion with 24 hours of live basketball. Even though it was 10 a.m. I got to watch Clemson beat the living tar out of Liberty University (a.k.a. Jerry Falwell University.) I take my joy whenever it presents itself so watching the Liberty student body endure this ass-whopping on national TV made me happy; two steps short of giddy. Suffice to say I'm not a big fan of Liberty University and the ideas it stands for. You can graduate with a degree in biology without ever really learning about evolution, but the players could not escape a beating by the hands of a superior team. Maybe it was God's will that made Clemson taller, stronger, more athletic, and better at basketball. If God really loved the good folks at Falwell University, why didn't He guide at least a couple of three pointers into the back of the net? This would not be the last time I questioned God's motives in the larger scheme of things.

Not having any idea what the next few weeks would hold for me, I decided I really needed to talk to my boss about my situation. The School of Education faculty at Indiana University East is a small and very tightly knit group of professionals. I know it sounds like a cliché but we are a lovable, neurotic little family. I asked my Dean, Dr. Marilyn Watkins, if she had a minute to talk. I do not like knowing that the news I have is going to shock and upset people. It seems unfair to them but there was no way around it.

"I need to tell you something and it's not good news." I have no idea what went through her mind but I can guarantee it was not a tumor on my transplanted kidney. I explained what I knew about my situation as she listened. Obviously she was shocked and concerned. I am one of the "old timers" at IU East and, as such, I am responsible for managing several important programs. But on that day, Marilyn's concern was for me and my family. I held together until I said, "I'm not sure what's going to happen to my kids" at which point I broke down and cried. I hadn't let myself really *feel* this yet or at least I hadn't had the courage to ask the question, "What will happen to my family if I die?" For those first few days it was sort of like a symphony was performing in my head but all the musicians were playing different songs. There were so many thoughts, fears, and prayers all jumbled together. It was not easy getting any work done.

A few days after the MRI I received the news that there were no indications of other tumors in surrounding organs. Whew! That was excellent news and surprising given the size of the mass. When tumors get really big they usually spread to other organs. I recently had the opportunity to tell one of my doctors this story and he told me, "You need to go out right now and buy a lottery ticket because you are the luckiest man in Indiana." This thing, whatever it was, was probably not going to kill me or at least it wasn't going to kill me in the next few months. The next step was to schedule an appointment with a surgeon. I contacted my kidney doctor (nephrologist) and asked for a referral which he happily supplied. As soon as possible, I set up an appointment with Dr. Little.

IS THERE A DOCTOR
IN THE HOUSE?

In early November my wife and I found ourselves in Dr. Little's office hoping for some kind of miracle. His surgical specialty is kidneys. Perfect. That's exactly what I needed. He looked over my copy of the MRI and made a few notes. He explained that the real question was whether he could remove the tumor and still leave me with enough kidney function to keep me off dialysis. What he really wanted was to see the disc containing the results of the MRI. That seemed like a logical request and we left his office charged with the task of getting a copy of the MRI disc to Dr. Little. We drove home to Richmond and took the request down to the folks at Reid Hospital. They explained that it would take a few days for the disc to reach Dr. Little.

What happened next was very strange and, to this day, I have no explanation. We never heard from Dr. Little again. Days went by as we tried not to jump out of our seats every time the phone rang. Days turned into weeks and eventually my brother called asking, "What's going on?" I explained that I couldn't get a hold of Dr. Little. My wife and I had been calling his office but he had not returned a phone call. We had no idea about the treatment plan. His nurse was exceptionally nice and I could tell she understood our anxiety. All she would ever say would be something like, "Dr. Little will be in surgery all day and can't take a phone call." She told both my wife and I that he had the disc because she had put it into his hand. My brother, Jim, who tends to be a bit emotional at times, was so pissed you could almost see steam coming out of the phone receiver. He advised

9

me in no uncertain terms to call Dr. Little's office and fire him. Jim said, "I wouldn't let a jerk like that within twenty feet of me with a scalpel." The next day I called Dr. Little's office and asked the nurse to deliver a message to the good doctor. "Tell Dr. Little he is fired. He is no longer my doctor." I thanked her for her courteousness during our interactions and hung up.

The next day I called my nephrologist and told him I needed another referral since Dr. Little was no longer my doctor. Almost a month had passed waiting for Dr. Little to get back to us so if he wasn't willing or able to do the job, we needed someone who could. A secretary called a few days later with the contact information for a Dr. Scott and we set up an appointment.

We met Dr. Scott a few weeks later and he seemed like a very nice man and dedicated doctor but something just didn't seem right. I could just feel it. My hunch was confirmed when the first thing out of his mouth during our consultation was that he wanted to consult with Dr. Little! I told Dr. Scott I wanted nothing to do with the man. We had come to see Dr. Scott after a frustrating month waiting for Dr. Little to communicate with us. I saw no point in forbidding Dr. Scott from discussing my case with Dr. Little but it was very clear from our interaction that Dr. Scott was not "the man." Dr. Little was clearly the head honcho but he was also either not able to help or not interested so I was back to square one. Later that afternoon I got a phone message from Dr. Scott saying that he had talked to Dr. Little and they both agreed that to remove the tumor they were going to have to take out the kidney. This was the news we had feared all along. Needless to say, we were devastated.

After mulling things over for a couple of days I decided I still lacked confidence in the diagnosis. Damn it. I wanted a third opinion! Obviously I wanted this "thing" out of me and I was aware that just because this tumor had not spread up to this point there was no guarantee that it would not spread in the future. So time was definitely of the essence. I also knew I wanted every opportunity possible to stay off dialysis.

AND NOW THEY GIVE ME THE ROTO-ROOTER TREATMENT

We need to back up for a minute and get back to my liver. That's where this story started and we are in danger of losing the plot. In the midst of all the drama with the tumor, there were still concerns that something was very wrong with my liver. I had seen my local gastrointestinal (GI) doctor and he said that what I really needed was an Endoscopic Retrograde Cholangiopancreatography (ERCP). When I asked him when we could schedule that he explained that the state of Indiana had a facility that is known throughout the United States for their work involving the ERCP. University Hospital in Indianapolis did more ERCPs than any hospital in the world. The main man over at IU Hospital was a guy named Stewart Sherman and he was the doctor I needed to see. My wife and I met Dr. Sherman, who is a short, intense-looking man with a great head of un-kept hair, and an ERCP was scheduled. (From here on out Dr. Sherman will be known as the Sherminator for no other reason than it made my wife and I giggle like school children every time we'd say it.)

During an ERCP doctors put a probe down your throat, through your stomach and liver, and into your bile ducts. Years ago I was diagnosed with a very serious liver condition known as primary sclerosing conlangitis (PSC) which is induced by a narrowing of the bile ducts. The bile ducts develop strictures inhibiting the flow of bile causing it to back up into the liver. This excess of bile in the liver can lead to infection and liver damage. In some cases, it leads to complete liver failure and death. Walter Payton, the former running back for the Chicago Bears, died of PSC.

My wife and I got up at the crack of dawn to make our way to Indianapolis for the ERCP. We headed to the pre-operative holding area, which was actually very comfortable. As I mentioned earlier, this place did more ERCPs than any facility in the world so it is safe to say they have the coordination down to a science. The various nurses and anesthesiologist came in to check on me. An IV was started through which I would get the happy medicine. The Sherminator eventually appeared and I was wheeled down to the room where he would play plumber with my insides. There seemed to be too many people in the room for a routine procedure but that's okay because I like being the center of attention. The anesthesiologist was a very large doctor who appeared to be in his early thirties. As they started to put me under he told me a story.

"When I was younger I used to be a caddy and I had the chance to carry the bag for the Dalai Lama. Big hitter, the Dalai Lama. He told me that on my death bed I will have total consciousness," said the doctor.

At this point I could feel the meds pulling me away so I said, "Doc, you have to talk faster. I'm going. . .," and immediately lost the battle for consciousness. I realized later he was repeating dialogue from the classic movie *Caddy Shack*. I'm sure lots of patients are scared witless prior to a procedure so he would tell them a story to distract them as they drifted off.

I woke up a couple of hours later feeling like I had been run through the wringer. The nurse asked me how I felt and I said, "My legs hurt." My legs felt exactly like they feel after I've had a muscle cramp. I couldn't imagine why my legs would hurt but they did. The anesthesiologist stopped by to check on me and I immediately said, "So finish your story about the Dalai Lama."

He smiled and said, "That was from *Caddy Shack*."

"I know," I croaked.

"How do you feel?" he asked.

"My legs really hurt," I told him. "It feels like I've had cramps."

"Well, you have had cramps. We used a medicine that produces extreme muscle relaxation and one of the side effects is muscle soreness like you've had cramping." Okay, I guess we've solved that mystery.

My throat was very sore, too. Ramming a tube down there certainly might have something to do with that. I was still very groggy but they wheeled me back to my little private area to be reunited with my wife. As I laid there sucking on ice chips and trying to shake off the effects of the drugs I came to another realization: I had shit myself.

Apparently the drug for extreme muscle relaxation isn't very discriminating. It works on *all* muscles. I wonder what it smelled like in the operating room. I hope it stunk. I wish I had eaten a dozen burritos the night before and washed them down with cheap beer.

I explained my dilemma to my nurse who was more than willing to clean me up. "Oh, no. That won't be necessary. I can handle that myself but I need to know where I can go."

She was not thrilled with the idea because I was still slightly loopy from the drugs but I convinced her and she led me to a small bathroom. She waited just outside the bathroom the entire time to make certain I didn't need assistance. I think she was afraid I'd fall but I was fine. Twenty-seven wet wipes later I emerged with a small portion of my dignity. I know I have no reason to be embarrassed but I was. It's funny how we all have our issues and having a nurse clean me after I messed myself was just too much.

Later, the Sherminator came in with pictures of my insides. One of my bile ducts was completely blocked but that didn't really surprise me because they had tried this same procedure twenty years ago and were unable to dilate one of my bile ducts. It was closed. It had probably been closed for twenty years. What I saw in the pictures he brought shocked me. He had inserted a very small stint in the closed bile duct. This stint was a temporary measure designed to help open the clogged duct. This stint also meant I'd have to have the same procedure a week later to get it out! It's a good thing the meds had worn off because I almost shit myself…again!

I thought, "Are you serious? I have to go through this again?" I couldn't believe it. Total price tag for the procedure: $14,000. So a week later, we hit "replay" and went to the hospital for another ERCP. Let me say for the record, I was not in a good mood but what choice did I have? That stint had to come out and there was only one way to accomplish that. The Shermintor had to go in and fetch it.

The parade of doctors started again. I was tempted to answer every question by saying, "You asked me the same question last week. Go back and see what I said then because the answer hasn't changed." But I didn't. When I met with the anesthesiologist this time I had a very simple request. I asked him, "What's the name of the drug that causes extreme muscle relaxation?" He immediately rattled off the name of the drug. I asked, "Do you have to use that again because I was sore as hell for about five days last time I had it." He assured me that he didn't need to use that drug and had no intention of giving me that medicine today. Inside, my bowels smiled. The chances of me pooping myself again were significantly reduced.

The procedure went much better the second time. The Sherminator called it a "home run" and said things couldn't have gone better. He also showed me the pictures on my newly dilated bile duct. They all seemed very pleased that they had been able to pry this thing open. I was pleased they wouldn't be screwing around with my insides for the foreseeable future. I still had a freakin' giant tumor in my belly and it was getting to be high time that somebody did something about that. Total bill for ERCP, part deux = $17,000.

TIME TO CHANGE TEAMS

A few days after things calmed down from my ERCP it was time to make some decisions regarding the tumor. Both Dr. Little and Dr. Scott were physicians at Methodist Hospital. The Sherminator was affiliated with University Hospital. Though only separated by a few miles, the difference between the two facilities was profound. I wanted to be cared for by the folks at IU Hospital. The Sherimnator was an amazing man and I had a tremendous amount of confidence in him and the rest of Team Sherminator. He is one of the only doctors I've had that would actually call or email me to answer my questions. My brother doesn't count. I had the Sherminator's personal email and if I had a question he would respond usually within a few hours. Maybe I'm a sucker for the personal touch, but that impressed the hell out of me. While I had no idea what type of doctor I needed at IU Hospital, I knew the Sherminator would know so I emailed him and asked if he would be willing to make a referral to a doctor who could help me with my problem. A few hours later he emailed back to tell me he had made a referral to Dr. Foster.

The time was now early December so it had been six or seven weeks since the tumor was accidentally discovered and I was not one bit closer to a treatment plan. I was now going to delay things even longer by deciding to go for a third opinion. I'm quite certain some people thought I was just delaying the inevitable but those people had never been on dialysis. If there was one chance to make it through this ring of fire without the end result

15

being dialysis, I wanted to explore that option. I was willing to go that extra mile because I would not want to second-guess myself later.

A few weeks later my wife and I were in Dr. Foster's office. I don't know the details but it was obvious the good folks working in the department that day had been experiencing what most people would refer to as a crappy day. The appointments were running way behind. When I go in for appointment I fully expect to wait 15 to 30 minutes past the scheduled time before being called. This day it was more than an hour. When we finally met Dr. Foster he apologized profusely and confirmed what I already suspected. Murphy's law was running roughshod over the urology department that day. There was no time for small talk. He asked the standard opening question, "What can I do for your folks today?"

I looked him in the eye and said, "I need a miracle. I've had two doctors from Methodist tell me that this tumor can't be removed without taking out my kidney. I'm here because I'm not 100% confident in that diagnosis so I'm hoping against hope you've got some better news." We had a brief discussion where I recounted my adventures with Drs. Little and Scott. He said, "It sounds like those guys didn't really know what to do with you and weren't too interested in figuring it out."

He asked if I had brought the disc containing the images from my MRI. I handed him the envelope with the CD and he excused himself to go examine the images. I knew the decision reached by Dr. Foster would probably confirm the treatment I would follow. Those few minutes seemed like an eternity when he suddenly stepped back into the room.

"Wow that is quite a tumor. Have you seen it?" he asked.

"No, we've never seen the MRI images," I answered.

"Come with me and I'll show you what we're dealing with," he said as he led us to a bank of computers. He brought up a series of images and there it was. At first I didn't understand what I was looking at but he helped Polly and I grasp the sheer magnitude of the situation. The tumor was absolutely massive. To novices like us, it's hard to appreciate how big a now 12 cm tumor (yes, it appeared to be growing) is but when you finally see it attached to my kidney, it made me sick. I was slightly weak in the knees as I looked at the screen. The tumor was so big that initially I mistook the kidney for the tumor. This damn tumor was bigger than my kidney or at least it appeared that way on the screen.

We headed back to his office to talk. He said, "Look folks, I don't think there is any way to save your kidney. It's going to have to come out."

I asked, "So there's no way you can leave enough of the kidney to leave me with adequate kidney functioning?"

"No, I don't see any way that will be possible. The other thing is once a tumor gets above 4 cm, they tend to leave behind little cancers even if you excise the existing tumors. We know that from autopsies over the years. So, once it gets above 4 cm we almost always remove everything because the cancer will come back if we don't," he explained.

Though not the kind I wanted, this sure as hell was closure. I felt a wide range of emotions in a very short period of time. An immediate sense of dread overwhelmed me. I was screwed. I might be able to survive this but I wasn't going to survive it without going back on dialysis. If it weren't for my wife and kids I can honestly say I would have spent some time seriously thinking whether or not I was willing to go back on dialysis. That would not have been an open and shut decision if I didn't have a family. Forty-eight years is a pretty good run. Maybe it's better to go out like this than to go back on dialysis. When I was in Dr. Little's office he told me a story about a patient of his who was in a similar situation. This guy chose death over dialysis. That might seem crazy to some but not to a former dialysis patient.

Dread soon gave way to fear. This thing very well could kill me and there was no way around that realization anymore. Hell, I watched a lot of people die slow miserable deaths on dialysis and that was twenty years ago. I had been told by several doctors, "Dialysis has improved a lot since you were on it last time," but I didn't believe that for a second. Things get better in medicine because people figure out how to make money improving the drugs or treatments. There were no fortunes to be made trying to help the poor bastards dying on dialysis. Who would be willing to devote their careers to helping dialysis patients? You don't get the key to the executive washroom by extending the lives of sick and dying patients. It's better to invent a new miracle drug or refine a surgical procedure that makes it available to twice as many people. That's how you make a name for yourself and land the big grants.

Dr. Foster was all business now. He was still way behind so he quickly transitioned into the next phase of the treatment: the surgery. "I think I would want to open you up midline," he explained as he motioned downward around my abdomen. He paused for a second and said, "You know maybe I should talk to someone in the transplant office. They may want me to do the surgery in a certain way that wouldn't interfere with anything they might do if you get a chance at another transplant. Who knows? Maybe you've got some incredibly rare condition I'm not familiar with," he said as he left to make a phone call to the transplant office.

While he was gone, my wife and I tried to put on brave faces. "Well, at least now we know what has to happen," I said and then tried to deflect some of the emotional energy of the situation by bashing Dr. Little. "Can you believe Little gave us all this runaround when he had to know the protocol for tumors larger than 4 cm? What an ass. Why would be screw us around like that?" I still have no answer for that question. We were each trying to wrap our minds around the implications of a return trip to dialysis. This is what we had feared and now it was here, hanging in the very air of the room with us.

Dr. Foster reappeared, gave a small smile, and said, "I'm glad I called them. They think you might have something called post-transplant lymphoproliferative disorder." I barely heard what Dr. Foster said because I was shut down at this point.

"What's that?" Polly asked.

"Well, it's a condition that sometimes occurs in transplant patients. A mass starts growing on the transplanted kidney," he explained. Dr. Foster then uttered a sentence that will be forever etched on my brain.

"If that is what this is, it's very treatable with medicine."

It took a second for my brain to process what my ears had just heard. "What did you just say?" I asked him.

"If it is PTLD then it is usually treatable with medicine" he repeated.

I was still having a hard time grasping what he was telling us. "By medicine do you just mean…medicine," I asked.

"Yes, it would be an oral medication," he responded.

As you might imagine, our moods improved considerably. I said to him, "I told you when I came here I was looking for a miracle and this qualifies."

He shook his head and said, "I didn't do anything."

"Oh yes you did. You knew enough to make a phone call," I said.

"Well, I really didn't do anything," he maintained.

"So what's the next step?" I asked.

"You need a biopsy to confirm the diagnosis and we can get that set up in the next few days," said Dr. Foster. "I'll have someone call you as soon as we've got a time for you."

We left walking about three feet off the ground. I knew there was a chance that this wasn't PTLD but at least there was hope. There was still a chance that I might escape from this relatively unscathed except for a sexy scar. It was a very good weekend at the Wildehouse.

HOLD STILL WHILE WE STAB THE SHIT OUT OF YOU

As my brother had predicted several months ago, there was only one way to know with 100% certainty if this massive tumor was, in fact, cancerous. Although all signs would suggest that it was cancer, I still needed a biopsy. If the diagnosis came back that I had PTLD then I wanted to start on whatever medicine I needed. Of course, I was well aware that the diagnosis could come back as cancer. I was sick of not knowing. Let's get this figured out. What the hell is this thing?

If any of you dear readers have had the misfortune of being "shanked" in prison then you've had a close approximation of what it's like to have a biopsy. The biggest difference is that with a biopsy, the instruments have been sterilized. I had a liver biopsy years ago and it felt a lot like being punched in the ribs if the person doing the punching was holding a small knife.

I arrived for the biopsy ready for the surgical stabbing. The procedure room was tiny. It was made to seem even smaller when the room filled with five people to perform the biopsy. First, the nurse got me prepped and explained the basics about what was going to happen. Next, one of the doctors came in and introduced himself as Dr. T but said I could also call him Dr. George. He had mercifully shortened his very long name that had approximately 17 vowels in it. I made it my personal challenge to call him by his correct surname. I asked him where he went to school and he told me the

University of Illinois. I ask almost every doctor that question in hopes I will run into a graduate from the University of Iowa. I'm still waiting. Go Hawks!

Dr. T's job included numbing me up with copious amounts of lidocaine. He started injecting me with a very long needle at the location where they'd conduct the biopsy which happened to be just below my belly button. The injections were painful at first. Anyone who has had lidocaine can tell you it burns like hell until you get numb. Deeper and deeper he'd go until he was confident I wouldn't feel anything from my waist down for a week to ten days. Then the real fun started.

Another doctor showed up along with a technician who was going to provide immediate feedback by microscopically analyzing the tissue they recovered from the biopsy. At first I thought they were telling me that they would know right then and there if this was cancer but they clarified that his job was to look under the microscope and make sure they were getting good samples that contained cells and not just fatty tissue. The room was so packed that his cart had to be out in the hall.

Dr. T was up first. He picked up his probe and I remember thinking, "That is the biggest damn needle I have ever seen in my life." I learned a long time ago that it's better to watch what doctors are doing to me than to wait for the pain. Well, I quickly abandoned that premise. Dr. T was very gentle and was kind enough to keep talking while he was stabbing the shit out of me. He used five or six hollow needles and then it was time for his partner who I'll call Dr. Stabs-a-lot.

As gentle as Dr. T was, Dr. Stabs-a-lot was the complete opposite. He probed me like he was enjoying it. Maybe he was getting paid by the thrust? It was ridiculous. I then did a very stupid thing. I asked, "Why do you two do this so differently? One of you is very slow and controlled and the other does it very rapidly?" I quickly realized this was a very dumb move on my part. That's like asking two economists a question about the effects of the deficit. There was an awkward pause in the room until Dr. Stabs-a-lot said, "It's a question of how you think you'll get the best sample."

"Oh, I see. Hey, who here likes the show *House*?" I asked hoping to distract two people with giant needles in their hands. Maybe this has been a point of contention between them. Maybe it had been simmering for years. Perhaps my question would be the final straw that pushed one of them over the edge (excuse the mixed metaphor) and they would decide to settle it once and for all right here in this closet. Thankfully, everything was cool and my faux pas didn't cost anyone his life.

After they had each stabbed the shit out of me with very long needles multiple times they turned to the lab tech. He was furiously trying to determine if the multiple stabbings were yielding good results. His verdict: not so much. They were getting a lot of tissue but it was mostly fat.

They decided to bring out the big guns (read "big knives"). They had these contraptions that looked like ice picks with plastic handles. The needles were just as long but hollow which was a better way of gathering core samples. Doc Stabs explained that they'd jab this thing into me and then, on the count of three, pull a little triggering mechanism to capture whatever was within the needle. It also made a horrible "snapping" sound so it was decided they should let me hear the thing on a trial run before putting it into my belly. Actually, that was a good idea because the sound is none too comforting. Sounded like a rattrap closing. So, just for shits and giggles, they stabbed me with six of those things. All in all, they took over twenty samples from my tumor but, as they kept saying, the worst scenario would be to find out that they didn't get a good sample and we'd have no choice but to do this all over again. They gave me a band-aid and I limped out of that damn closet.

AND THE VERDICT IS…

The days following the biopsy were horrible. There was no escaping the realization that within a few days I would know whether I had cancer or somehow I had lucked out and this was just a harmless growth. Even though I went to work, taught my classes, and tried to carry on like everything was normal, inside I was a mess.

I was at the computer a few days later checking my email when I saw that there was an email from Dr. Foster. "This is it," I said to myself and opened the email. I was scanning the email so fast I couldn't find the answer to the $64,000 question: Is this cancer? I re-read the email and figured out why I was confused. Dr. Foster had left out the one word that would answer the question. His email said, "*Your biopsy showed only necrosis (dead tissue), ossification (aberrant bone formation), and atrophic tubules (shrunked normal kidney). It is definitely not   Necrosis and ossification can occur in renal cell carcinoma, so the kidney should probably be removed. I talked to Dr. Bill Goggins who is the main renal transplant surgeon here, and we think you would be served best by having him remove the kidney, since he will be the one to determine when you receive another.*"

The phrase, "It's definitely not…" seemed incomplete. Definitely not what? Cancer? PTLD? I quickly emailed him back saying, "I think there's a word missing in your email. I'm not sure what you mean." Of course, after I sent my email I could do nothing other than sit at the computer and wait for a reply. I'd hit the "Send/Recv" tab every two seconds. He emailed back a couple of hours later apologizing for his mistake. He clarified, "Yes, it is cancer." Shit. I put my head down on the desk and cried.

So months after the ultrasound determined I had a large mass on my kidney, I finally get the official diagnosis...cancer. Now there is no longer a question about the treatment options. There is only one...remove the cancerous growth, and with it, my only kidney.

HEY PAL, COULD I INTEREST YOU IN A CATHETER?

Once it became apparent that I was going to be on dialysis, there was work to be done. There are certain preparations necessary to make dialysis possible. There was very little time because once they removed my kidney, I would have to start immediately.

There are two kinds of dialysis: peritoneal and hemodialysis. Peritoneal dialysis is performed by having a catheter inserted into your peritoneal cavity (abdomen). The catheter is used to allow fluids to be pumped into the cavity, held for a period of time, and then drained out. The process uses your peritoneal wall as a membrane across which fluids and dissolved substances (electrolytes, urea, glucose, and albumin) can be removed from the blood. It's a little like washing your socks in the sink. The water is clean until you put in the socks. After awhile you drain out the dirty water, put in clean, and wash the socks again.

I was on peritoneal dialysis for about ten months the first time my kidneys failed back in the early 1990s. It was a disaster. The advantage of peritoneal dialysis is that it is designed to do the exchanges automatically while you sleep. That's the plan anyway. Imagine trying to sleep while fluids are being pumped in and out of your belly all night. The damn alarm would ring when the machine malfunctioned which was fairly common. Not only was I exhausted from not sleeping, I wasn't getting enough "clearance," which is a fancy way of saying I was swimming in toxins. I tried peritoneal dialysis after spending months on hemodialysis because I wanted to be able to do my treatments at home rather than spending three evenings a week hooked up to a dialysis machine in Milwaukee. Eventually I had no choice but to go back to hemodialysis. I can't ever remember being sicker than the time I was on peritoneal dialysis.

So when I knew I was going to need dialysis again, it was an easy choice. Give me hemo or give me death! But there was a slight complication. Hemodialysis is performed by directly cleansing the blood which is usually accessed by placing needles into your arm. The needles are inserted into something called a fistula which is created by surgically fusing a vein with an artery. The vein then has increased blood flow which helps with dialysis. My problem was that there wasn't time to create a fistula. I had a fistula years ago when I was on dialysis but it had stopped working. The recovery time after surgically creating a fistula is about six to eight weeks. The only option now was to put a catheter into my chest which would lead directly into a chamber in my heart. Hemodialysis could then be performed by accessing my blood through this catheter. Sounds fun! I'm sure you're wondering where you could get one of those.

So on Friday, February 19th (three days before the surgery to remove my kidney) they put a catheter into my chest. When they explained that the catheter would be going into a chamber of my heart, I was a little concerned. My heart is one of the only organ systems that still seemed to be functioning as designed. I don't like anybody messing around with my ticker but this had to be done.

I always try to remember that what seems like a big deal to patients is routine for doctors. They probably put in three of these things before lunch. The docs and nurses were very nice and reassured me that this was a routine procedure. So they put me under conscious sedation and jacked a catheter into my left chest. No big deal. I remember coming to with AC/DC playing on the radio which seemed appropriate since February 19th is the anniversary of their former singer's death. R.I.P Bon Scott.

On the ride home I kept touching my chest and thinking, "Wow! This thing is permanent." I got home and looked at it in the mirror. Ewww! Gross. It's like your mind says, "That's not supposed to be there." But it was there. Get used to it, mind.

I was about to become a dialysis patient once again and my life was going to change. The Dialysis Union, Local 142, tried to trademark the phrase "Abandon all hope ye who enter here," but apparently it was already spoken for. You've got a tube hanging out of your chest? Big deal. You've been split open, had an organ taken out? Ho-hum. Your veins and arteries will be stitched together? Yeah, that too. Wait until you get to see the unit where you'll be hooked up to machine to keep alive. It's to die for! Price tag for one catheter: $7392. (A bargain if you ask me.)

TIME FOR A NEW SCAR

Our worst fears were realized. I needed surgery to remove a very large, cancerous tumor on my transplanted kidney. There was no way to save the kidney so I would enter the operating theatre with normal kidney functioning and leave without it. Dialysis…here I come.

The surgery was scheduled but in the weeks leading up to it, I was determined to have so much fun that if I died on the table it would take the mortician two weeks to get the smile off my face. And at the Wildehouse, fun is spelled ICE CREAM!

I'll admit that I have a few weaknesses. After all, I am not made of steel. The white substance known as cocaine is of no interest to me. Why would people give away all their money so they could go to a hotel room and sweat for three days while their testicles shrink? Count me out. But the white substance known as vanilla ice cream…different story. If there were a 12-step program for ice cream abuse I'd be a member. "I admit I am powerless over ice cream." I would be on a "no ice cream" diet for quite a while so I decided to see how much of it I could eat in the days prior to the surgery. The answer was "a lot." When I checked in for surgery I was close to 200 pounds which is more than I've ever weighed in my life. My thoughts were "mission accomplished" because I knew the weight would fall off me once I was back on dialysis.

I don't remember much about the days leading up to the surgery other than I was trying with all my might to keep a brave face for everyone. Truth be told, I was scared shitless. Most people heading into a major surgery are worried about the procedure. That wasn't me. I wasn't the least bit concerned about the surgery. How hard could it be to cut out a kidney? Plus, this kidney was just below the skin in my lower abdomen….piece of cake to get that thing out. I was concerned about surviving on dialysis long enough to have another chance at a transplant. Dialysis absolutely sucks and I was headed back to that life. In all honesty, I was ambivalent about living and dying. I didn't want to die but it wouldn't have been such a tragedy if the surgeon screwed up and I croaked on the table. However, I knew that wasn't going to happen. No way I'd get that lucky.

The day of the surgery started at an ungodly hour. We were up and out of the door around 4:30 a.m. Polly and I decided to bring the kids along. At first I was hesitant because my instincts are always to shield them as much as I can from the bad stuff in life. Polly thought otherwise and, as usual, she was right. I wanted them to have as normal a day as possible which would still be very abnormal with their Dad headed to surgery. Still, I'd rather have them sitting in school, distracted, not learning, and surrounded by their friends than in a hospital with me. Polly thought that was a terrible message to send to them. We're a family. We're in this together and we support each other through good times and bad. So over to Indianapolis we all drove through the darkness. The tension in the car was so thick you could have cut it with a knife. I remember we listened to Bob and Tom on the radio, trying to be distracted as best we could.

Once we checked in I had an acting job to do. I had come down with a cold over the weekend and I was afraid they were going to postpone the surgery. My thinking was that the surgery was inevitable, let's get it over with. I'm here. Let's go. Let's do this thing. I was able to convince the various docs that my cold was no big deal and, as it turned out, it was a baby cold anyway. We played my favorite game of 50,000 questions again. They started me on the IV and took me back to a room to get ready. I asked if my family could come back and they did. Once again, I tried to reassure them it was going to be okay. My son, Jack, was worried about the surgery. I told him that a trained chimpanzee could remove a kidney. At some point they put this metallic looking cap on me that was shaped like a pouffed chef's hat. I had Anna, our daughter, take a picture on our cell phone. A few weeks later Polly said she hated that picture because it reminded her of such a horrible time in our lives. Duh! I should know better than to do stuff like that but I was born with a clown's soul. I always, but always, go for the laugh. I hate to see my family uptight and worried. Solution: delete the picture from the phone.

Off to surgery we go after a delay of about ninety minutes. Polly's sister, Sally, had taken a day off of work to be with the family, which was great. Polly and Sally are very close and I know my wife really appreciated the support. I'm going to skip the description of the surgery because I was there but, obviously, out like a light. I have a few fuzzy memories of later on that day.

Our minister, Eldon Harzman and his wife, Sharon, were in my room at one point that day. I was still pretty out of it because they give you the really good drugs when they are going to cut you open like a Christmas goose. The drugs were working really well because I had no kidney function to pee out the meds. They were just simmering around in me. How cool is it that my minister came all the way over to Indianapolis to be with my family during our time of need? To this day I think of that whenever I see Eldon or Sharon. I have never been a big fan of organized religion but that doesn't change the fact that I love my church family. They have been, and continue to be, a source of strength through all this. Massive props to the members of Central United Methodist in Richmond, Indiana. My church family kicks ass.

Polly and the kids left in the late afternoon and a few weeks later she told me she felt terrible about leaving me there in that condition. My wife is a worrier and she can dream up things to be concerned about that would never occur to me. She was afraid some evil nurse would poison me because I was too sick to do anything. Okay. That would rank slightly below "being hit by a meteorite" on my list of things to worry about.

That first night was a strange one. I kept pumping my pain button as often as I could. I'm no hero. My alarms kept ringing all the time. The poor guy in the room with me probably got no sleep. I kept saying, "Sorry brother," and he'd call over, "Don't worry about it." I was so out of it I couldn't tell the difference between his alarm and mine. I'd apologize when his alarm rang, too.

I'm going to be honest and say that I have no memories of the day after surgery other than when I had my first dialysis treatment. They wheeled me down a couple of floors, hooked me up via my catheter, did treatment for a few hours, and wheeled me back to my room. That's it. Nothing traumatic but then again, I was in the hospital. Who cares what is happening to you while you're in the hospital? It makes no difference to me if I am in a bed in my room or in a bed in the dialysis center.

Now the third day got a little more interesting. The day started very early, like they always do in the hospital, with my surgeon and his team coming in to check on me. They looked over my incision and decided it was time to take off the flimsy excuse for a bandage. I got my first look at my incision and the word that came to me mind was "impressive." That baby was about ten inches long and did the neatest curve around my belly button. Now I try to show it off as often as possible. My surgeon, Dr. Goggins, had some news for me regarding my tumor. Turns out it wasn't renal cell carcinoma as everyone had suspected. It was clear cell carcinoma, which was great news. This meant that I would not be required to wait several years for a transplant. When people are diagnosed with most forms of cancer, another transplant isn't even considered until at least two years have passed. If there happen to be any cancerous cells remaining in the body, these cells would go crazy when the immune system is suppressed following a transplant. There would be nothing to fight their growth so the protocol for transplant after cancer is at least a two-year wait.

Polly arrived a few minutes after the docs left. The kids were back in school and Aunt Sally had gone home so it was just Polly this time. She asked, "Have the doctors been in yet?"

"Oh yeah, I forgot to tell you. They were just in and I didn't have renal cell carcinoma," I explained.

Her eyes focused on me with the expressions of both anger and curiosity. Anger as in, "How in the hell could you not tell me this news?" and curiosity as in, "What kind of cancer was it?"

I continued, "I have something called clear cell carcinoma which is apparently good. Dr. Goggins called it a 'bullshit cancer.' He said that if you have to get a cancer this is the kind you want to get."

Polly was obviously pleased at this news but not fully comprehending the implications. "So what does that mean about another transplant?"

"It means I don't have to wait. I can go on the transplant list fairly soon. Dr. Goggins told me a story about a guy who had clear cell carcinoma last November. He removed the guy's cancerous kidney and transplanted a new one during the same operation," I explained.

At that, Polly started crying. And when I say she started crying I mean she *really* started crying. She cried and cried and cried. She cried so long and hard that I could hear the people in the room on the other side of the curtain getting quiet. I realized they had no idea what was going on so I told them, "It's okay folks. It's good news, not bad. My wife is happy."

So up we went on the never-ending emotional rollercoaster. As I've figured out by now, you should never get too high or too low. What we didn't realize at the time is that it is one thing to be eligible for a transplant. It is another thing entirely to have a matching kidney available. You can be on the transplant list but without a matching kidney, what good does it do you? Oh, and the average wait time in the great state of Indiana for an A+ positive kidney is two and a half to three years. So our elation eventually became tempered when we found out that little nugget of information. Still, I'd much rather be the survivor of clear cell carcinoma than any of the other types. The docs aren't worried about the cancer spreading so I guess it means I will make fewer visits to the doctor's office over the long run. I kept reminding myself, "This is great news." Oh really? It doesn't feel so great.

I wish I could recall more details of my hospital visit but I can't. The days after surgery were pretty boring. Wake up, try to eat, take a walk around the floor, back to bed, go to dialysis, back to bed, talk to some friends/family, back to bed, try to eat, take another walk, back to bed, call it a day.

After four days, they let me go home. I was excited to get home and watch my Iowa Hawkeyes take on the Northwestern Wildcats in basketball. I got situated for the game but I was so out of it I could hardly pay attention to the TV. That's okay because Iowa played terribly and for all intents and purposes the game was over after ten minutes. I had strange voices running through my head. There were times I wasn't sure where I was. I felt like death on a stick but I guess when you feel crappy, you might as well feel that way at home in your own bed. So, I was home but good God, what was my life going to be like now? I kept repeating, "We've just got to get through the next two months. Things will get better if I can make it through the first two months." In retrospect, I was absolutely right but I don't think I anticipated how difficult the first couple of months were going to be.

I wish I could tell you what all the various charges added up to for my little adventure in the hospital but that's very difficult to track down. I can tell you it cost $12,453.25 to use their very nice operating room. The recovery room services came in at $1652 while radiology services were merely $1263.25. Thank goodness I have insurance or I'd be looking at getting a second job.

AND DIALYSIS IS HER NAME

Most people on dialysis lose their kidney function through a slow, insidious process. For some it takes decades from the time when they were made aware they had some type of problem until they reach a point where their damaged kidneys are not giving them enough clearance. At that point, dialysis is the only choice if they want to keep living.

My first experience with kidney disease and dialysis followed that course. I was made aware that I had End Stage Renal Disease (ESRD) from a routine physical but much of the damage had already been done. I had only 18% kidney functioning left. There was very little the doctors could do to prolong the life of my poor, sick kidneys. I was on dialysis within a few months.

This time, I wound up on dialysis through the "express lane." Rather than going from zero to 100, I went from 100 to zero in an instant. I entered the operating theatre with 100% kidney function and left with 0%. And once you are on dialysis, there is no honeymoon period. You can't "rest up after surgery" and take on dialysis when you are feeling better. You'll be dead. That remains true for days when dialysis patients have medical procedures. There are no days off from dialysis. Three days a week...regardless. That should be on a sign outside of each and every dialysis center in the world. You had a colonoscopy today? Too bad...get your ass in the chair. You had a root canal? Tough titties... get your ass in the chair. Your catheter got infected and they pulled it out of your chest and stuck in a new one? So sad... get your ass in the chair. You caught your wife bonking the plumber? I feel for you...get your ass in the chair. You caught your husband bonking the plumber? Here's a quarter, call someone who cares and… get your ass in the chair. It seems cruel but that is life to a dialysis patient. Only death is an escape.

The weekend before I had my surgery the family went on a hunt for the local dialysis center. I really wanted to know where the place was before I started. I had a general idea of the location of the place and I double-checked it in the phone book. When we got to the address, it was apparent that this was not a functioning dialysis center. In fact, the building looked like it was empty. I happened to look across the street and there it was (insert angelic music here), the Fresienius Dialysis Center in Richmond, Indiana. Rather than just be happy I had found the place, I was intent on going in and saying hello. Even though it was a Saturday afternoon, the place was open and doing business. There wasn't a receptionist on duty so we peered into the room where patients were getting dialysis until someone noticed us and came over. Her name was Kim and, as it turned out, she would be my nurse for most of my treatments for the first few months. Having people like Kim around you is one of the reasons dialysis is tolerable. She has fire-red hair and genuinely cares what happens to her patients. You might think that attitude by the nursing staff would be universal but that would be a mistake. To some of the nurses and techs, we cease being people and become "the work." We are not fathers, husbands, grandmas, aunts and uncles. We are patients, nothing more, nothing less. Our problems become their problems and, truth be told, we have a lot of issues. Our catheters don't work. We get infections. We bleed and puke all over the place. We scream out in pain from massive body cramps brought on by dehydration. In the end, we make their days harder. I always had the feeling that some of the staff gets pissed at us for being sick. I am happy to say I spent many evenings in Kim's care and I never, ever felt that way. She treated me with the utmost dignity and care.

So on the first afternoon of my treatments I arrived at the dialysis center feeling lower than I can ever remember feeling. This was exactly the scenario I was trying to avoid. This was the one thing I did not want to endure. Obviously, dying would stink (not to mention ruining your weekend) but at least you wouldn't have to endure dialysis. But here I was and, yes, I will whine to you, dear readers. I was not going to be a whiner to my fellow dialysis patients. Everyone suffers but you do it in silence. Man up and take it.

I had no idea what to do because the set up was quite different than when I was on dialysis in Milwaukee back in the early 1990s. They called my name and I entered the inner sanctum. At this facility, no one was allowed beyond the locked door other than dialysis patients and staff. No friends, family, or anyone not giving or receiving treatment. They weighed me, took my temperature, and escorted me to my assigned barcalounger.

One thing I noticed immediately was that I didn't have any "stuff." As I surveyed the unit I noticed everyone else had tons of blankets, cell phones, books, magazines, grills, blenders, golf clubs (okay I am exaggerating but I was amazed at the amount of accoutrements people had.) Actually, that made perfect sense. Anything to pass the time and make the stay less boring and more normal is a good idea. I walked in with nothing.

When patients start dialysis there is a certain amount of guessing that occurs regarding our "dry weight" which is the weight we have immediately after dialysis before we've gained pounds by drinking. Since most dialysis patients don't make urine (or make very little), our weight fluctuates dramatically based on how much we drink. For example, my buddy Henry recently gained thirty pounds between Monday morning and Tuesday evening. That is not a typo. He gained thirty pounds!

Part of dialysis is to remove the excess fluid that accumulates between treatments. The good folks at the hospital were nice enough to send over an approximate dry weight to the people at the dialysis center. There was only one problem. The dry weight from the hospital was figured with me in a robe and nothing much else. When I arrived at the dialysis center in Richmond I was wearing a full set of clothes, shoes, wallet, and all the other articles of modern life. What that meant is they were going to suck fluid out of me until they got me down my weight in the hospital. Big problem! A person's clothes, shoes, etc. probably weigh somewhere between 5-7 pounds. They were now planning to take off those 5-7 pounds from my fluids, which would leave me a quart low so to speak. When people get dehydrated, they don't feel so well. I was about to experience that first hand.

The first three hours of dialysis went fine. I kept pinching myself to make sure I wasn't having a nightmare. I wasn't. This was all too real. The last hour of dialysis is when they pull off the fluid and about 20 minutes into this hour I started to feel funny. My hands started to tingle. I had no idea what this meant so I didn't bother to tell any of the nurses. I kept feeling worse and worse as the hour wore on but I was being too tough to say anything. I finally mentioned I was feeling rather poorly and by that time it was too late. I was zapped of fluid like a vampire had just had his way with me. I was sucked dry. At the very end of the treatment they always want to get your sitting and standing blood pressure. That was a problem because I was so dizzy from dehydration I couldn't stand. They held me up and got a BP of 75/45. Lovely! No wonder I felt like crap.

One of the nurses asked me, "Do you think you can walk?" "No," was the obvious answer. Truth be told I'm not sure I could have crawled out of that place. I took comfort in the fact that I was positioned in a barcalounger that allowed me to see into the waiting room. There was my beautiful wife waiting to take me away from this madness. They wheel chaired me to the scale, took my weight, and I headed home. "The first one is always the toughest," I said trying to convince myself as the world spun in circles around me on the ride home. I'll be back, day after tomorrow, to "get my ass in the chair" again. This cycle will keep repeating until one of two things happens; I get a transplant or I die. Three days a week…regardless. That really should be an actual sign on the wall.

FUN WITH FISTULAS

I mentioned earlier that I had to have surgery to get a fistula. As I sit here tonight, I am hooked up to the machine through a central line catheter that has an arterial and venous port. These two lines merge into a central line (thus the name central line catheter) that gets lodged into the upper chamber of my heart. Yes, I am writing this with a catheter stuck into my heart. As would be expected, this is not a good long-term solution. Catheters fail from time to time but the real danger is an infection that could be very serious given the fact that this tube is directly connected to my ticker. By "serious" I mean fatal. But really, most dialysis patients aren't that scared of the idea of death. We're already half dead. For some, kicking the bucket would be welcome release.

The better permanent solution to the central catheter is a fistula created by a surgical procedure where a vein is fused with an artery. My first fistula was almost twenty years ago but I can remember it quite like it was yesterday. I hadn't been fed through the teeth of the medical machine yet so any type of medical procedure was a big deal. Back in 1990 my fistula was done under local anesthesia. The anesthesiologist was a younger man who came in and immediately started chatting with me. Hey, I always appreciate the effort. Obviously people are shitting their pants (in this case, my gown) and most doctors make no effort to try and help the patient relax. This gas passer was the exception.

He asked me, "Mr. Wilde, do you like music?"

I said, "Actually, yes, I love music."

"What kind of music do you listen to?" my new best friend asked.

That's always a bit of a sensitive subject because my tastes are unusual. I am 48-years-old and I still love metal! Always have, always will. I am drawn to a genre of music known as "doom" which originated with Black Sabbath. Some of my favorite bands are groups no one has ever heard of unless you're a 19-year-old Scandinavian metalhead. I answered his question in a somewhat safer way not wanting my new best friend to reject me on the basis of my love for Swedish doom metal. "I like hard rock," I said.

"Have you ever heard of a band called Deep Purple?" he asked.

Have I heard of Deep Purple? Are you kidding me? What self-respecting metalhead hasn't heard of the Purple? Not one of my all time favorites but still a great, great band that is still going strong.

"I love Deep Purple," I replied with enthusiasm as I started to be aware they were cutting on my left wrist. It didn't hurt because of the meds but I knew they weren't over there trying to steal my watch.

We went on to have a discussion of our favorite DP albums. One of my favorite guitarists is a guy named Tommy Bolin who did one album with Deep Purple in 1975, *Come Taste the Band*. He had the impossible task of trying to replace the original guitarist Ritchie Blackmore. Tommy's contribution to the DP catalog has been sadly overlooked by many so I tried to convince the anesthesiologist to check out *Come Taste the Band*. Before I knew it, I was wheeled out of the room and into recovery. My fistula worked like a champ for the entire time I was on dialysis.

Fast forward twenty years: I was in need of a new fistula. Sometimes fistulas keep functioning even when the patient is no longer using them but sometimes they just stop. Mine quit when I was out on a run. The docs had prepared me that it will probably just stop working one day. By "stop working" what I mean is the "thrill will be gone." Fistulas create an unnatural amount of blood flow through the vein, since it is fused with an artery. There is a buzzing or thrill in the vein that you can feel and even hear. I can hear mine if I sleep with my wrist near my head.

I was given a referral to a local surgeon to have the procedure done. This time it would have to be up near my bicep because the veins and arteries used for my first fistula were compromised. I talked it over with my brother and asked, "Should I make it an appointment to see a specialist for this or is a local guy good enough?"

Jim said, "Well about 30% of these things fail so I'd think about going to a surgeon who specializes in this type of procedure." That was all I needed to hear. I asked the dialysis doctor who swings through once a month if he could recommend someone and he immediately said, "Dr. Sheridan, he works on our most difficult cases. I've sent three or four people to him that other doctors said that there couldn't be fistula put in and he was able to do it."

I scheduled an appointment with Dr. Sheridan whose office is in the northern part of Indianapolis about ninety minutes from my home in Richmond. Prior to the surgical procedure an ultrasound was used to analyze the veins in my arm. The results of the ultrasound indicated that the veins in my bicep were fine and the procedure was scheduled for a Wednesday. Since I have dialysis on Wednesday the surgery was going to be first thing in the morning (or whenever the surgeon arrived.) My wife and I got up at 4:00 a.m. to get to the hospital on time. We went through the typical day of surgery song and dance. My favorite is the 50,000 questions game usually played by at least two nurses.

One change from twenty years ago was that the procedure would be done under general anesthesia (GA) which sucked because that made five GAs I'd experienced in about 75 days. I asked the anesthesiologist (who made no effort to be my best friend) when they made the shift from local to general and he said, "A lot of it depends on surgeon's preference" and that's probably true but I also know that the price of the GA probably topped what the entire procedure cost last time. So they give me the sleepy meds and, boom, I was out like a light.

The next thing I remember was waking up in recovery wet with sweat. Eventually they got some dry gowns on me and I made it back to my little recovery area to be with my wife. She explained that she had talked to Dr. Sheridan who told her, "Things did not go as planned." Huh? They did the surgery (I could tell because my arm was starting to hurt.) "What didn't go as planned?" I thought through my drug-addled mind. Soon after that Dr. Sheridan appeared and explained that the "vein was not what they had hoped for" which seemed odd since everything had looked fine from the vein mapping they did with the ultrasound.

I've been around long enough to know when I'm being let down easy. When your girlfriend is trying to become your ex-girlfriend, she usually starts the conversation with something like, "I've been thinking about our relationship and I think we're strong enough to date other people. It might even strengthen our relationship." She doesn't start with, "My feelings of contempt for you are such that I can no longer contain them. I absolutely hate you. Die you bastard die!" She'll let you down easy because it's easier on everyone involved.

Dr. Sheridan was giving me the preamble to his version of a break-up talk. It's easier if you start by saying, "Things may not work out so well." That allows for some hope, even if it is diminished. I went to see Dr. Sheridan a couple of weeks after my surgery. He listened to my new fistula (which is as quiet as a Quaker church) and officially pronounced the fistula "dead." And then we made other plans. They can keep the catheter in my heart but do I want to do that? Hell no. They may have to start carving up my right arm. I don't like either of these options but those are the choices before me. I just can't seem to catch a break. So in the end, all I got was another scar, a very large bill headed to my insurance company, and the promise of another long, shitty day in the hospital.

DON'T LET THE DISEASE DEFINE YOU

A phrase heard quite often when dealing with chronic illness is, "Don't let the disease define you." The logic behind such a saying makes a lot of sense. Patients would do better if they focused on the areas of their lives that remain largely intact despite their illness. I started thinking about that on one of my drives over to dialysis and I realized that pithy little phrases are easy to say and a lot harder to live by.

I wake up in the morning and feel an immediate, overwhelming sense of exhaustion. As a dialysis patient, I'm learning, again, to live without much sleep – as it is a precious commodity these nights. Last night I slept from 10 to 11 p.m. and then woke up hard. The waking up is never gradual. I wake up irritated, itchy, and jealous of the person in bed next to me happily sawing logs. I managed to drift off to sleep again about 3:30 a.m. and slept until about 6:30 a.m. A total of four hours of sleep is about average. I have had nights where I literally do not sleep for one minute and I still have to stagger out of bed and go to work.

So after I get my wits about me I realize that my mouth tastes like a cat has shit in it. That's not a fair comparison because I've never actually had a cat do its business in my mouth. However, it does taste terrible. It's a sickly sweet taste *that never goes away*. I brush my mouth until my gums bleed knowing full well that the taste will return like a bad penny in about twenty minutes and be with me the rest of the day.

I go downstairs and contemplate breakfast. There's not much I can eat. I settle on an apple because I know apples are low in potassium and phosphorus; two things I have to constantly watch in my diet. I've been eating bushels of apples the last couple of months. Oh, and just for the record, Ben Franklin was full of it. An apple a day does not keep the doctor away.

I get to work and it is a glorious day where I am employed. I am a college professor and today is the day when our senior students turn in their portfolios. This is a huge deal for them. They have worked countless hours on their projects. They are in a raucous mood and it quickly spreads to the faculty. A couple of students stop in to say, "Hi."

"Dr. Wilde, we're having a party down in room 310. We have lots of food. Would you like to stop by and get something to eat?" Judy asks.

"Well, that depends. What kind of food do you have?" I respond.

"We've got cookies?" Judy says.

"What kind are they?" I ask.

"Chocolate chip and they are homemade. I think Donna made them," she says with a smile.

I make a pained face, "I can't have chocolate."

"We've got chips."

"Nope, too much salt and phosphorus."

"There are cup cakes but they're chocolate too," Judy offers.

"Too bad because I love cupcakes," I say.

"We've got cheese sticks," she says hopefully.

"I can't have any dairy," I shrug.

I decide to go down and be sociable by spending a little time with the students. I wasn't really hungry, anyway. I look over the spread of food and, sure enough, there was literally nothing there I could eat on my diet. I took three crackers back to my office and tried to scrape the salt off.

It's now close to time for class. Mercifully, I have a small group to contend with today. Only twenty students and the semester is drawing to a close. As I look back at my teaching since the surgery, I have had to make some significant adjustments. I just don't have the energy to teach the way I would prefer. It may not seem like it but to teach a class for three and one half hours is exhausting. I've struggled trying to find the energy I need to do my job the way I am accustomed. I've had to turn over more of the instruction to short group projects where students think and discuss various topics. While this is a useful instructional tool, I've gone to "the well" too many times with this technique this spring. I am doing this because these short breaks give me a few moments to rest. I make it through class. It was an okay session but I am plagued by the memories of how I used to teach this content. I know I can do better and that is a painful realization. This is my life's work and it is way too important to do it badly.

Lunch time rolls around and I have a scrumptious selection packed from home. Some type of beef (chopped sirloin perhaps) and white rice. Of course there are no additives or flavorings to bring out any taste in the food. That's actually not such a big deal because there is very little joy left in eating. Remember I'm swallowing this through the cat shit filter. A student stops in to ask some questions while I'm trying to choke down my food and apologizes profusely for interrupting my meal. I tell her she's doing me a favor.

This is an early day for me so I make it home around 1:30 p.m. I'm exhausted and would love to take a nap but I'm not sure that's in the cards today. I've got several projects around the house that I need to attend to and if I don't do them now I'm not sure when they will get done. After a brief internal struggle I say, "screw the projects" and climb into bed. I can usually drift off to sleep relatively quickly and I do. I am out like a light and the next ninety minutes are the best part of the day. Sleep, glorious sleep. I wake up feeling disoriented. Is it morning or afternoon? I realize my kids will be home soon so I make my way downstairs for the all too brief time I will spend with them that day. They get home about 3:30 p.m. so I have one hour to do my day's worth of fathering before it is time to head off to dialysis. That hour always goes too fast and before I know it I'm leaving. There's usually only time to get them a snack, talk a little about their day, and make sure they get started on their homework.

It's 4:30 p.m. Time to dance with the devil. I will arrive home after my 4 ½ hour shift close to 10 p.m. and I will be completely spent. I feel like a juice box that's been stomped on by a fat kid. I am also famished so I pile down whatever food my long suffering wife has prepared. I eat and immediately head to bed as I can do little else. That first hour of sleep after dialysis is deep but I know I will awaken and have to figure out what to do with myself for most of the night. Like I said earlier, sleep is a precious commodity. You take it whenever you can get it.

Prior to my illness my wife and I enjoyed a very healthy (and active) sex life. That thought makes me chuckle aloud as I type it. There is nothing healthy (or active) about it now. When we do have sex, it is often used medicinally. "Maybe it will help me sleep," is part of the thought process. Passionate? Nope. Vigorous? Please. I think my wife deserves a medal for even making the effort.

So all in all, I think I'm doing a fairly good job of not letting the disease define me. It only affects every aspect of nearly everything I do. But the struggle continues. I will not relinquish this life without a fight. Right now the best I can do is to keep breathing and listen for the lessons to reveal themselves.

DON'T WORRY,
I'M JUST BLEEDING

For the first two months, I was bounced from chair to chair within the dialysis unit. I made projections that within four months I would be in every station in the facility. Then, all of a sudden, I was placed in the same chair for a couple of weeks. As luck would have it, I was right next to Bruce.

Bruce has been on dialysis for about a year. He ended up here as the result of testicular cancer. He had been diagnosed with a kidney disease years ago (some type of polycystic disorder) but his kidneys had been functioning perfectly...until the radiation treatment. The doctors maintain that his sudden (almost immediate) kidney decline had nothing to do with the radiation therapy. Bruce thinks differently.

"How could my kidneys be just fine one day and then, in the course of a couple of days, fail completely?" he asked. He has an excellent point. It makes no sense for kidney functioning to implode unless there was some outside factor influencing that decline.

Something happened to Bruce a few nights ago that shocked me and I can't seem to get it out of my head. It was right at the end of his shift which had been uneventful. The nurse removed his needles. After they remove the needles, you have to put direct pressure on the wounds for quite a long time to make sure the bleeding stops. The way the veins and arteries of dialysis patients have been surgically modified, causes a massive amount of blood flowing through those veins. The doctors and nurses drill it into your head that if you somehow manage to sever that vein, you need to get a tourniquet on it immediately or else you could bleed out in about ninety seconds.

Bruce is holding gauze on his wounds for at least ten minutes and is just about ready to be bandaged up and sent home. All of a sudden, blood starts pouring out of his arm. The gauze had become completely saturated and at that point, blood flows through the gauze rather than stopping the bleeding. The blood is flowing out of his arm like a faucet and a very large pool is forming at his feet. The pool is getting bigger with each passing second.

Bruce calls to a nurse, "Hey, I need some help here" but he did it in a very calm voice. The nurse didn't even hear him. I've never been shy and I get extremely un-shy when a friend of mine is leaking blood like a sieve. So I yell, "HELP!" at the top of my lungs. Several of the nurses in the area and turned to see what the shouting is about.

One of the nurses responsible for Bruce sees the blood pouring out of him and very calmly strolls over. Her pace is not one bit faster than if she were walking over to shut off one of the alarms that ring incessantly. Quite frankly, I am stunned. Obviously the nurses who work in a dialysis unit are up to their asses in blood. They are desensitized to it. They work in blood the way a baker works in flour. Also, looking back on the situation, it was clear that Bruce was not in any real danger. We were in a unit with numerous nurses and techs. He had direct pressure on his wounds so it was just a matter of getting some fresh gauze on him. However, did any of the nurses think about the message being sent to the other patients? It couldn't have been any clearer if they had printed it on t-shirts. Even when blood is flowing out of you, they're not worried. By the end of this ordeal, there was a puddle of blood about 12-15 inches around. It looked like a scene from a TV detective show.

So fifteen minutes later, Bruce is headed out the door to his family. The blood is cleaned up and everything is fine again. It's hard to wipe that image from my mind. What's even harder to forget is the indifference I saw that night. It does not leave me with a great deal of faith in the people who keep me alive with these machines. I'm asking myself, "What would it take to get these nurses to actually quicken their steps?" I hope to God I never find out.

ARE THOSE REALLY *MY* BUTT CHEEKS?

The changes to my body over the past few months since the surgery have been rather remarkable. I've lost more than thirty pounds in the three months since I checked into the hospital to have my kidney removed. When I look in the mirror, the physical changes are apparent but we all know that images can be deceiving. Those mirrors are designed to make us look thin. Sometimes what we need is tangible proof. You know, evidence we can feel.

Like the other night when I was in bed and my butt itched. I reached around to scratch it but quickly became distracted by the shape of my very own butt. It felt…wrong. It felt…foreign. Whose butt is this anyway? It felt like I was scratching the butt of a 20-year-old version of me. Weird. I look in the mirror and sometimes I'm not quite sure who's looking back.

Losing weight on dialysis is not something I try to do. It just happens. To start with, I feel sick almost all the time. I say "almost" because there's a short period of time after dialysis when I feel just about normal. The rest of the time I feel pretty crappy. Who wants to eat when they feel sick? It's just not something that is enjoyable so it's easy to skip.

One thing that is different from the first time I was on dialysis is the puking or lack thereof. When I was on dialysis in the early 1990s I vomited on a regular basis. So regular, in fact, that we kept paper grocery bags stashed all over the house because I couldn't tell when I was going to vomit. All of a sudden, I'd just puke. When most people are going to vomit, they know it.

There are the warning signs that we all know. I felt so lousy all the time that I couldn't read those signals.

So unlike my last experience with dialysis, my weight loss cannot be attributed to regular upchucking. The main reason weight falls off me when I'm on dialysis is because of the diet that I'm required to follow. Dialysis does about $1/7^{th}$ of what a kidney can do. It filters off some of the impurities and removes excessive fluid but there's a whole bunch of stuff in that other $6/7^{th}$ that is essential for good health. For example, dialysis can't regulate the body's levels of phosphorus and potassium. The only way to manage those levels is to follow the dialysis diet. Basically, the dialysis diet could be renamed the "If it Tastes Good, Spit it Out" diet. It's pretty restrictive. Here are a few of the things you have to go without on the dialysis diet.

1. Dairy — Dairy products are very high in phosphorus and if your phosphorus levels get too high, you run into problems. The first problem is that your skin itches like crazy. You can't stop itching to the point of causing lesions on your skin from excessive scratching. Try sleeping when you itch from head to toe. My wife has told me that I can actually scratch myself in my sleep but then again, I've always been special. The other minor issue you run into with high levels of phosphorus is that your internal organs start to calcify. Now I'm not a doctor, but having a calcified heart doesn't sound good. I'd like to avoid that if possible.

   The problem is, though, that diary encompasses about 90% of all the really good stuff to eat in the world. Bye-bye, ice cream. Imagine living without ever having the ability to wrap your lips around a bowl of Neapolitan or plain old vanilla. It sucks! Dairy also includes things like…milk. Try eating your Fruit Loops dry sometime and let me know how that works out for you. Actually you can use non-dairy milk as a substitute and that's not completely awful. You know the non-dairy creamer people put in their coffee? That's what we get instead of milk. Again, it's not great, but it is passable.

See ya later butter! Margarine is the next best thing and, oh my, I **can** believe it's not butter. Sometimes a slab of butter is just better than margarine but, truth be told, I can manage this one pretty well. My wife doesn't like having to use margarine when she cooks, though.

Cheese. That's right, no cheese. Keep in mind I grew up in the shadow of Wisconsin which makes living a cheese-less life even more sad and pathetic. Cheese makes everything better. How did we manage to choke down our veggies as kids? Cover them in cheese and anything is edible. You could cover an old textbook in cheese and I'd be tempted to take a nibble. Our family went to a "pitch in" (or "pot luck" for some of you) at our daughter's high school a little while ago. Everyone brings some food to share and usually people bring one of their best dishes (which is why these things are great). I could barely find anything I could eat because everything had cheese in it. There were 27 varieties of macaroni and cheese and, had I been able, I would have tried them all. Benjamin Franklin said, "Beer is proof that God loves us and wants us to be happy." I'd like to extend that to cheese as well.

Of course, cheese is an essential ingredient in the greatest food that has ever existed: pizza! When a man has pizza in his life, he can tolerate almost any indignity. No matter what life throws at him, he can manage because he knows at the end of the day there is pizza. Imagine life without pizza. It's not a pretty picture, is it? When you've reached an important milestone in your life and you want to go out and celebrate, you don't celebrate with burgers. You don't party with spaghetti. You go out for pizza with your friends and family to mark the occasion. That's just how it is.

Our family has a routine where every Friday night we have pizza. We might have had pizza Monday, Tuesday, and Thursday of that week but when Friday rolls around and pizza is not on the menu, there is a problem. Friday is pizza night. No excuses. I have been somewhat lucky because on Friday nights when my family is in full-on-pizza-orgy-mode, I am at dialysis and blissfully unaware of the carnage taking place at my home.

2. Potatoes — Keep in mind the dozens of different forms the almighty potato can take (all of them delicious, too.) Who doesn't love burying their face in a bag of chips every once in a while? No more French fries. See ya later tater tots. Hold the sour cream and butter on that baked potato. Better yet, hold the baked potato. Do you think Thanksgiving would be incomplete without a pile of mashed potatoes? You do? Well, tough titties because if you were on dialysis, you'd have to find a way to celebrate the greatest football holiday known to mankind without mashed spuds.

3. Chocolate — No, I am not kidding. No chocolate. Please take a minute and let that sink in. Ladies, take two minutes. No more chocolate chip cookies. Brownies…bye bye! Forget about all your favorite candy bars. Milky Way, Snickers, Hershey Bar, The 100 Grand Bar, all of them…gone. That big slice of chocolate birthday cake with a side of ice cream…not gonna happen. Life without chocolate is a life not worth living. Well, get used to it.

4. Bananas — Perhaps not a big deal for some but when bananas become the forbidden fruit, they seem like the greatest thing in the world. Man, I miss bananas. If I ever get a transplant I'm going King Kong and eating a half dozen in one sitting followed by a loaf of banana bread (with butter) and a giant glass of milk.

Bananas are high in potassium. As I mentioned earlier, dialysis doesn't do a good job of regulating potassium. Too much potassium and your heart stops. So potassium is not something you want to "cheat on" your diet. Having said that, I think a majority of dialysis patients think of the dialysis diet as more of a recommendation than something they absolutely need to follow. I get the sense from many of my dialysis brothers and sisters that they know their time is short so, what the heck? They're going to eat whatever they want with the time they have remaining on this earth.

5. Pop (a.k.a. soda) —Now you can have some kinds of pop but none of the good kinds. Pepsi, Coke…gone. Sprite and 7-Up…yes. That's not a fair trade. There are very few things I was addicted to but Diet Mt. Dew was one of them. I should have bought stock in the company I drank so much of that stuff. It was basically all I drank. Now I'm cold turkey on the good stuff and politely sipping away at a Sprite just because it has slightly more taste than water. Ugh!

Even if I was able to drink the good stuff, I wouldn't be able to drink very much of it. Dialysis patients have to be very careful regarding the amount of fluid they drink because we don't have the ability to pee it out. So we do things like chew gum to distract us from the fact that we are *thirsty*. I really miss guzzling pop.

So you see, who couldn't lose weight with a diet like this? If you follow it, you are going to lose weight. I remember telling some of the people I work with that if I had to go back on dialysis I'd lose between thirty and forty pounds. I could tell they thought I was crazy. I didn't think it would happen quite this quickly but I knew I'd lose a lot of weight.

The rapid changes to my physical body have been shocking but not nearly as surprising as the changes to me…the real me, my inner self, or whatever you want to call it. Right now I want you all to feel really sad for all of us dialysis patients. I'd like you all to acknowledge those feelings by scarfing down a bag of chips, a banana split, and a dozen Hersey Kisses. A finer tribute could never be paid.

THERE'S SOMETHING
ABOUT SARAH

Have I told you about Sarah? She runs the same shift as I do (Monday, Wednesday, and Fridays from 5 – 9:30 p.m.) We're usually the last two coming off the machines at night but that's not why I'm writing about her. Actually, I'm not exactly sure why I am drawn to Sarah but, the fact is, she invades my consciousness on a regular basis whether I am at dialysis or elsewhere.

It's always really hard to guess a dialysis patient's age because this unnatural process ages us rapidly. But if I had to guess Sarah's age I'd say somewhere between 55 and 60. She has piercing blue eyes that always brighten a little bit when we talk. When I really contemplate why I think about Sarah so much the answer is pretty simple. She's very sick and each dialysis treatment is an exercise in suffering for Sarah. I sit and I watch her suffer and I feel hopeless and sad and pissed off and I want to grab God by the collar and shake the shit out of Him. Why? What did this poor woman ever do to deserve this? And if you are Master and Commander of the Universe, why aren't You helping her?

I'm not the most religious man you're ever going to meet but my wife and I both want our children raised in the church so they have that foundation. If they decided later on that organized religion isn't for them, well, at least they've had the proper exposure. I feel lost at church and often wonder why I am attending. It is a rare occurrence when I feel anything of a spiritual experience while I'm lip-synching from the Methodist hymnal. But when I'm in dialysis, I pray hard. I pray like if I do it the right way maybe, just maybe, I can help remove some of Sarah's suffering. I ask God to give her suffering to me. I'm stronger and I could bear her burden. I don't think God is listening.

Sarah went through a stretch a few weeks ago where she was feeling very nauseous and vomited during every treatment. I don't care who you are or what your claim to fame might be, I defy anyone to look cool puking while sitting in a recliner. You have to sort of arch your back and try to project the vomit into a little receptacle. Some patients puke and then, five minutes later, feel much better. That doesn't seem to be the case with Sarah. She gets sick and stays sick. Sarah often moans when she's not feeling well and I feel helpless and pissed off all over again.

The nausea is just a minor issue for Sarah. She also has periods when her blood pressure is dangerously low. How low? Like 90/45 low. It's so low that she's on the verge of being unconscious. Her right foot doesn't look good. I'm not sure but she may be diabetic.

When I look at Sarah, I try not to see a dialysis patient. I try to see a child of God. In fact, even though I just finished telling you I'd like to grab God by the collar and shake Him, it is also at these times I feel like I am in the presence of God. I am stuck with the same question philosophers have been wrestling with for all of recorded history. Why must people suffer? Why must Sarah have a body that is falling apart on her? I go out of my way to talk to her. I want to tell her I'm praying for her but, somehow, that doesn't seem right. I don't know why. I imagine one of these nights it will pop out. I have no idea how she'll react which is why I keep that thought to myself.

I want for Sarah what I want for everyone: life and life abundantly. The "abundantly" part means I'll gladly take the good with the bad because that's all part of the nature of this existence. I want the lawn mowing. Bring it on. I want baseball games…all kinds. I love them all. I want more long hugs from my daughter. Even though she's sixteen and I have been anticipating the separating process for some time now, she still treats me as though she's happy to have me around. Go figure. If I didn't know better, I'd swear she's five instead of sixteen. Either we're doing something right or her behavior is dictated by feelings of guilt and fear that I might die on her. Either way, I'll take it. Give me more movies and music and sex and all the things that make life worth living. Heck, give me the stuff that makes life a pain in the ass, too. That's part of what I want and I want the same things for Sarah. I don't know if either of us has a chance to find the more abundant life but I guess that's not important. What is important is to take notice of these small interactions. Honor the pain by being fully present when it hits you or affects a brother or sister in dialysis.

Viktor Frankl wrote about suffering after he survived the Nazi concentration camps. He believed that suffering had purpose. In this case, people who are suffering with kidney failure gain a perspective that would be impossible without the struggle and pain, and, yes, the suffering. Frankl said, "*The truth--that love is the ultimate and the highest goal to which man can aspire. Then I grasped the meaning of the greatest secret that human poetry and human thought and belief have to impart: The salvation of man is through love and in love. I understood how a man who has nothing left in this world still may know bliss, be it only for a brief moment, in the contemplation of his beloved.*"

I love you Sarah and I will continue to worry about you but I think I get it now. All this time, I had been trying to save you. I had it backwards. You're the one who's been saving me.

MY BIGGEST ORGAN

I've been having all sorts of trouble with my biggest organ. I'm not sure what it is but something is just not right. For starters, it itches all the time. My wife spends half of her waking hours scratching it. Then there's the problem I have each morning. I wake up and my biggest organ is all tingly. Then after a few minutes, it starts to feel like bees are stinging it. Yup, there's definitely something wrong with my skin. Wait, what did you think I was talking about? Geez, get your mind out of the gutter. I thought everyone knew that skin was your biggest organ.

It's not just the skin, though. This whole ordeal is really starting to wear me down. I was thinking about it while I was hooked up to the machine and I realized that the exhausting part is that "it's always something." This illness just slowly chips away at your health…brick by brick. At first it was the overall shock to the system of having my kidney removed and having to go on dialysis. Eventually I gained some of my strength back and became a functional human being again. At least I was strong enough to go to work and stumble around in front of a class. Then it was the guessing game of dialysis. Trying to find my correct weight was nearly impossible as I was losing weight at such a staggering rate. A few weeks later the drama turned to an infected catheter, which was diagnosed after a trip to the emergency room. Shortly after that there was surgery on my arm to create a fistula. Of course, that failed so another surgery is being planned. It just never ends. It's rare that a week goes by without something new cropping up.

This illness reminds me a little bit of golf. The key to playing good golf is getting all phases of your game working at the same time. That almost never happens. One day you can drive the ball a mile but can't make a putt to save your life. Then you're putting like Jack Nicklaus but your short game is a shambles. Dialysis is a lot like that. There's always some type of drama, some issue just around the corner waiting to rear its ugly head. The latest drama for me is my biggest, baddest organ...my epileptic epidermis. Oh, how does my skin itch? Let me count the ways.

Well, for starters I just have your normal everyday itchy skin, which is no big deal. My skin is itchy probably because dialysis dries me out. I slather on lotions and oils and it seems to help a little or at least I'd like to believe it does. But lotion is no substitution for backrubs. The number one family activity at the Wildehouse is backrubs. At times we must seem like a group of monkeys sitting in a circle picking bugs off each other. A few months ago my daughter rubbed my back so hard I was bruised for a week. It felt awesome! But this type of itchy skin is just an annoyance. No big deal.

Next, we have the "oh-my-god-I'm-starting-to-sweat-and-I-feel like-I'm-being-stung-by-bees" itching. This one is no joke. As the name implies, it happens each and every day when I start to perspire. There's something very, very wrong with my skin. It is not normal to be in this kind of agony every time you start to sweat. And, yes, I do mean agony. On a scale of discomfort from 1-100, this is a 95. I try to do my best to attack this problem head on so I climb on the treadmill every damn day and try to get it over with as quickly as I can. It takes about 1.5 miles to get to the point where I no longer feel like ripping the flesh from my bones. I don't even bother to mention this problem to the doctors anymore because they tell me things like, "Try some Oil of Olay." This has got to be some type of nerve problem but it points to the bigger issue of the relative ineffectiveness of dialysis. People are born with kidneys. We do great with kidneys. When those little rascals no longer work, we have all sorts of trouble.

Now it may seem like these two types of itching would be enough fun for anyone's largest organ but no, the gods of dialysis had a meeting a few weeks ago and decided I needed even more fun in my life. My latest "organo mas grande" problem is the most bizarre. It happens each time I lie still for a couple of hours like after I sleep or have a dialysis treatment. After I wake up my hands and feet start to itch. If itchy had a measure like a seismograph, this type of irritation would be equivalent to the San Francisco earthquake of 1906. I literally cannot scratch fast enough or hard enough. If possible, I could use three sets of hands and still have a few places to scratch. This little beauty started a few weeks ago and has steadily been getting worse. Now it appears to be spreading up my legs rather than just being located in my feet. The last time I was on dialysis my feet went numb after about a year. What I wouldn't give to have a numb pair of feet now. It only lasts about fifteen minutes but still, what the heck? I can't even take a nap without having to suffer for it.

It's hard to describe how problems like these wear you down. They are a constant source of concern because they are always in the back of your mind. I have to consider the very real possibility that if I try to go to the post office I may start sweating which would cause me to completely freak out. The best way to deal with a "bees-all-over" attack is to take my shirt off. Well, the employees in the post office are nice but I'm not sure they want to see me shirtless in their establishment.

All of this is just exhausting and it definitely plays with my mind. I feel trapped knowing that each and every day these tiny tortures wait for me. I can do nothing without taking these conditions into account. I'm going to a football game on Saturday but I need to find time very early in the morning to get down to the treadmill so I can get through the "bees-all-over" attack so that I don't have to experience that in the stands surrounded by my family. They don't want to see that. Maybe if I could just get a little relief I'd handle this better but who am I kidding? There are no days off. And while I'd like to think I'm stronger than this, it makes the thought of death seem almost inviting. At least it would be a release from this...shit. But I have to stop thinking like that. When I get past all the bullshit I realize that when I start fantasizing about death that I'm really just being selfish. My family didn't sign on for this either. They don't deserve to be fatherless and widowed. My wife pledged "in sickness and in health" and she's holding up her end of the bargain. I need to endure this. I need to endure all this for Anna and Jack. Damn this would actually be a lot easier without them. Love and pain are two of the great paradoxes in life. The more you love, the greater the pain you will endure. Still, I guess it's worth it in the long run.

Now it's time to go climb on that treadmill and slay this fucking dragon again. I can take it. I don't have a choice.

BLOOD SCRUBBING IN
THE WITCHING HOUR

When I was first on dialysis roughly twenty years ago, I was scheduled for a 3 ½ hour run. It seemed like an eternity but what choice did I have? Spending 3 ½ hours in a chair three times a week was way better than spending eternity in a very expensive wooden box. After my surgery in February of 2010, I started back on dialysis with a 4 hour run. It may not seem like much but that extra thirty minutes was a problem for me. This was probably due to the fact that during those thirty minutes all I could do was say to myself, "I should be done now. I used to be done by this time. I could be driving home now." Weird but true. Those thirty minutes seemed a lot longer.

For some reason a four-hour run was insufficient. My labs were terrible and by "terrible" I mean like "unprecedented…world record… unheard of." One of the things the labs measure is the level of creatinine in your blood, which is one way to measure kidney function. People with normal kidney functioning should have a creatinine level of 1.0. Most dialysis patients should be around 3-5. My creatinine level was 16. When I told my brother the news he said, "I've never heard of anyone having a creatinine level of 16. I didn't know the scale went that high." Lovely. But like I've told you, I'm special.

Having an elevated creatinine level means my blood is filled with toxins. My blood contains all sorts of things that my kidneys should be filtering out. I thought to myself, "Perhaps this is why I feel so terrible." My dialysis was extended to 4 ½ hours in hopes of bringing down my creatinine. Again, that extra thirty minutes was akin to torture. After a few weeks, labs were drawn again. Drum roll please. My creatinine had dropped all the way to 13.8! Whoa! Things were headed in the right direction but not nearly fast enough. The doctor and staff started to mention a third option—nocturnal. A small number of patients actually do dialysis over night as a means of getting more dialysis. My immediate reaction was, "Not a freakin' chance." I envisioned myself trapped in the recliner, wide-awake surrounded by snoring/farting dialysis patients. I can't sleep in my own bed at home. How the heck am I going to sleep in a dialysis center?

I started to give the idea some serious thought. "Well," I said to myself. "I obviously need more dialysis and this seems like about the only way to get it. So what if I'm awake all night in a recliner. I'm awake all night now. Plus, I would be able to see more of Jack's baseball games and spend more time with the family." I decided that once school was over I would give it a try.

The night of my first nocturnal treatment was at hand and I was trying to wrap my head around the whole thing. "Remember, if I get more dialysis they tell me I'll feel better. Maybe if I feel better I could actually sleep like a human being." With fear and trepidation I showed up at 9:45 p.m. for a six hour (yikes!) run. One thing I liked right away was that the nurse, Trey, was waiting for me. During the daytime you have to sit in the waiting room for about ten minutes before someone comes to get you. Trey explained to me, "We do things a little different here. When you get here just go ahead and weigh yourself and take your temperature. Then head back to the corner. That's where you'll be." Cool. I can handle that.

There are only about eight or nine patients on nocturnal so it's a small crew. I have a feeling this nocturnal thing is something that you either love or hate. Some people swear by it. I'm willing to bet those are the people who can sleep.

The room is darker and much quieter. During daytime dialysis the cacophony of alarms and bells is deafening. They told me that they readjust the machines so the alarms don't ring as much. Again, cool. That works for me. I head back to the corner and realize that the recliners are gone and we have beds instead. That's a bonus because those beds aren't made out of plastic so there's a chance my ass won't fall completely asleep. Some air may actually reach my butt during this six-hour run.

So the nurses hook me up to the machine and the treatment gets started. Without warning all the lights in the room go off and something strange happens. Suddenly the dialysis center now resembles a trendy nightclub except there is no music or dancing or drinking or fun of any kind. But in some weird way it looks vaguely like a club with the colored lights on the machines and the glow of the televisions around the room. The sound of techno music is replaced by the hum of machines circulating blood. Simply put, I was slightly creeped out.

I'm sure this will come as a shock but I did not sleep at all during my first six-hour nocturnal run. It was the longest six hours of my life. It was even longer than the movie *Out of Africa* that went on forever. It probably seemed even longer because it was the first date Polly and I went on and all we wanted to do was get out of there and talk. Still, that damn movie just would not end.

There were times I was sleepy but I couldn't doze off. This might be because even though they change the way the alarms on the machines go off, they still make a hell of a lot of noise. So it went from deathly quiet to BEEP, BEEP, BEEP about every three minutes. This cycle repeated all night. Relaxing.

As an unexpected bonus, the guy in the bed to my left was having bad dreams. Every thirty minutes or so from midnight on he'd scream, "Momma! Momma! I didn't do it Momma." I kid you not. You couldn't make this stuff up.

Mercifully, the clock struck 4 a.m. and I slunk toward the door. I had a mantra in my brain, "Bed, Bed, Bed." I ate something and practically crawled up the stairs to sleep. I'm pretty sure my wife didn't sleep much that night either. She doesn't like being home at night without me. Even the dogs were upset. Our two dogs won't go upstairs to sleep in our bedroom until both Polly and I are in bed. This posed a problem for Myrna and Roscoe. They stayed downstairs all night waiting for me. Occasionally Roscoe would wander upstairs to see if I had somehow made it to bed. Now that's loyalty.

When the second night came around, I had a whole new plan. DRUGS! I asked the doctor if there was any way they could give me something just to knock me out. My brother said that was certainly a possibility. Obviously they have drugs that will do the trick and it wasn't like I needed to be doing anything during dialysis. I just needed to physically be there. As expected, my dialysis doctor didn't like that idea. He said, "Well, you have to be able to drive home afterward so we couldn't do that." I was irritated because driving home after dialysis is not an insurmountable problem. How about a cab? Maybe my wife could pick me up? Let me translate what the doctor was really saying: "Your comfort and general well-being really don't mean shit to me. I'm not going to make any effort, no matter how small, to help you feel better outside of a medical intervention. You can't sleep. You feel exhausted. I just don't care all that much. I only care about the numbers on your lab print out." Well, I can't say I was shocked. So I took matters into my own hands.

I have been experimenting with various over-the-counter meds and also with my left over pain medications. I've discovered that a combination of Benadryl and one pain pill has worked the best. It makes me drowsy and also relaxed. I don't feel so agitated. So around 11:30 p.m. on the second night I took my pills and tried to chill out. Then something magical happened. I slept. I slept for almost two hours! Un-freakin'-believable. I even had a dream but it was almost like a nightmare. I dreamed I was in dialysis at night and that I was sleeping. In my dream I made it all the way through dialysis to the end of the night and they had to wake me up to take me off the machine. I woke up and looked over at the clock and realized that I still had three hours of dialysis left. Major bummer! But still, just the idea that I could sleep made this nocturnal dialysis seem much more doable.

It has now been a little over a week in nocturnal and I'm hanging in there. The guy in the bed next to me keeps having bad dreams about his mother but that's alright. He seems like a delightful guy and I purchased earplugs that help quite a bit. They took my labs at the end of last week and told me my creatinine level was dropping which is the reason I'm doing nocturnal. I'm not sure I can do this shift once school starts up again in about a month but I'm getting used to it. Sometimes creepy nightclubs can be sort of cool.

THE ABSOLUTE BEST THINGS ABOUT HAVING A LIFE-THREATENING ILLNESS

I can probably guess what many of you are expecting me to write in this chapter. Something along the lines of, "The greatest 'gift' that comes along with illness is the new perspective about the little things in life." You know, the little things like a quiet meal with your family takes on new significance. You're expecting me to say I'll never take life for granted. Sorry. That's not true for me. You see, I was on dialysis for nearly two years so I gained that appreciation a long time ago. I've never lost it either. Every time I'd wake up at night and have to pee I would thank God. It was easy to remember the times when that fluid was being removed through very long needles stuck into my arm. I don't take the little things for granted. One of my favorite quotes is from Dostevsky who said, *"There is only one thing I dread: not to be worthy of my sufferings."* What is it about those Russian guys? They just know how to get to the heart of the matter.

Having a life threatening illness is no fun. In fact, it sucks. But I can't find anything positive about being constantly negative. It just doesn't help anyone. You've got to stay positive. It is with that sentiment in mind that I present this list. Here's my list of the best things about having a life-threatening illness.

1. My wife —I have an amazing partner. I know many of you think that your spouses are great and I'm sure they are fine people but, with

all due respect, my wife is better than your wife. I *know* I wouldn't have made it this far without Polly. She has been right by my side through all of this…all the procedures, all the tests, all the pain, all the surgeries. What most people don't realize is that she has the toughest job of all. She has to sit by the side of someone she loves, watch that person suffer, and know that there is not a damn thing she can do to prevent it. I have the easy part. All I have to do is be sick.

I've been trying to write this little tribute to her for a week. Actually I've been avoiding it because I know I won't be able to capture my feelings about Polly. Words fail me. I'm not nearly talented enough as a writer.

When I'm really feeling lousy, the only person who can help is Polly. When we are in bed and I can't sleep, I ask her to put a hand on me. Just having her touch on my shoulder or back relaxes me. I can feel my body begin to calm down. She is like a drug. And as I write this I know we have a lot more "stuff" to get through. More procedures, more tests, more surgeries. I know she'll be right there with me until the bitter end. And that, perhaps more than anything, makes me want to live.

2. Prayers — Lots of folks are praying for you and that can't hurt. I'm not convinced it does much good but the fact that people are consciously focused on my health is humbling. I have friends from years ago who have reached out with an email or phone call. How great is it to pick up the phone and it's an old college buddy you haven't heard from in ten years? I always feel better after that phone call. I always do if for no other reason than the reminiscing about past misdeeds. Trust me, if you knew the guys I went to school with you'd understand.

    Sometimes people avoid us "sickies" because it makes them feel uncomfortable. "I don't know what to say," is the standard line. The truth is you don't have to say much. Just let your friend know you're sorry they're not feeling well and ask, "Is there anything I can do?"

In general, just let them know you're thinking about them is all you need to say. Mission accomplished.

3. Pasta — There is no way I would have survived childhood without Kraft Macaroni and Cheese. Come to think of it, I probably wouldn't have survived graduate school either. Even though I miss a lot of my favorite foods, I still get the noodles and that's fine by me. But, please, hold the cheese for now.

4. Increased efficiency — I am at least 28% more efficient at work since I no longer have the need to take frequent restroom breaks. As a matter of fact, I no longer have the need to take any restroom breaks. While everyone else is running back and forth to the bathroom, I'm working away and getting lots of important things accomplished. I think I'll point this out to my boss and ask for a raise.

5. Slacking — Sometimes you can get out of stuff you don't want to do. You have to be careful not to abuse this one but every once in awhile you can play the "I'm not feeling well" card and get out of some chore. The thing about kidney failure is that, for the most part, we look normal. If friends need you to help them move to a new house, brothers and sisters, play that card! Play it and don't feel guilty. What kind of nerve they have to ask someone who is clearly on death's door to help them move? Selfish jerks! Please remember you have to save this one for special occasions. Don't waste it if your wife asks you to take out the garbage. Rookie mistake.

6. Weight loss — The weight just falls off you. So far I've lost around 35 pounds since my surgery. I'm starting to look like a heroin addict. Damn, I'm getting really skinny. And, I'm not trying to lose weight at all. Actually, I'm trying to stabilize and put some weight back on but obviously, that's not working. So if you're one of those people who have tried every diet and still can't lose weight, try the dialysis diet. Google it. If you follow it, I absolutely guarantee you that you'll lose a ton of weight.

7. Anticipation — This one is big because there are so many things we can't do, can't eat, and can't drink. We've already covered the "If it tastes good, spit it out" diet. There are so many simple things that folks with kidney functioning take for granted. I spend hours anticipating what I'm going to do if I'm lucky enough to get another kidney and I have several very elaborate plans. This is one of the little games I play in dialysis to pass the time. I asked my new best friend Bruce, "What are you looking forward to doing after you get a kidney? He said, "I want to drink an entire can of Coke and then I want to pee it out." See what I mean? He didn't say, "Take a vacation in Hawaii." He's looking forward to urinating. Not many people can say that.

8. A Whole New Set of Dreams — We dialysis patients have an entire new set of dreams to occupy our night time hours. I bet most of you never dream of a Hershey bar. How often do you dream about drinking a glass of milk? Not too often I'm willing to bet. Sure we still have the normal sex dreams and such but there's a whole new set of dreams just waiting to escape behind the walls of sleep. Yes, it's weird but it's also kind of wonderful.

9. Scars — I've heard it said that chicks dig scars and I really don't know if that's true. I've yet to ask a lady about her feelings on this issue. But I do know that I am very proud of my scars. I will show them off to anyone almost anytime. My scars are my battle wounds. They are signs of my trials and tribulations. They are a visual testament to the events that have shaped me. The suffering I have gone through has changed me and I'm confident that evolution is for the better. Plus, my scars look awesome. I am one sexy man.

Well, that's about it. Not much of a list I guess but when life gives you lemons, make lemonade, and then look forward to peeing it out. That's what dialysis patients do anyway.

A STRANGE THING HAPPENED WHILE I WAS GETTING MY BLOOD WASHED

It happens before each dialysis treatment. It's part of the routine. As the clock ticks closer to the time when I must leave my family, a certain sadness creeps in. Dialysis patients all get it. We *have* to go for this treatment. There really isn't a choice. Well, that's not entirely true. People skip treatments and we watch what happens to those people. They have a funny way of dying. We watch that and take mental notes. Lesson learned. Don't skip treatments.

June 15th, 2010 was a night like every other night. Everyone got weighed in and had our temperatures taken. We got our surgical masks in place before they stab us so we wouldn't get another infection. Some patients, like me, don't get the giant needles in the arm. Not yet anyway. They hook us up to the machine through a catheter. The catheter crowd avoids the pain of the needles but everything gets balanced out by the pain of an infected catheter.

But let's get back to the 15th of June. It was as normal as any other night. The alarms kept ringing. Blood pressures were either too high (mine) or too low (everyone else). The problem occurred after the witching hour. While the 15th was "same old, same old," the 16th was a tad more exciting.

The man who serves his time next to me is Henry. It's always hard to guess the age of a dialysis patient but my best estimate would be around 70. His hair and beard are as white as snow. Also, his tattoos are faded but, in all honesty, that could be attributable to a lousy tattoo artist. A lot of Henry's parts are missing. He has no toes on his left foot and only a couple remaining on his right. Similarly, he has several fingers missing on his right hand. I've been doing my treatments next to Henry in the nocturnal shift for a few weeks now so I don't know him well. I do know he is the noisiest sleeper in the world. He talks more in his sleep than most people do while awake. Henry also has recurring bad dreams regarding his mother. But all of that has nothing to do with the situation that made June 16th so unusual.

Around 2:00 a.m. I heard Henry babbling in his sleep. A short time later he appeared to be more awake and I heard him say something about "wetting the bed." This struck me as odd not because a grown man may have peed on himself. Those of us on the dialysis unit abandon all semblances of dignity and normal physical functioning. Anything and everything is possible here. Peeing on yourself? No big deal. What was unusual about the idea of Henry peeing on himself is that he's a dialysis patient and I could tell he was a long timer. I couldn't imagine how he was still making urine. That's what caught my attention. A long time dialysis patient peeing on himself just didn't make sense.

About that time the alarm on his machine went off and, believe me, there's nothing unusual about that. Those damn alarms ring constantly. Once I was talking to my brother during a treatment and there were so many alarms going off that he said, "It sounds like a circus down there." Trey came over and said, "What is going on over here?" Even in the dim light produced by the glow of dialysis machines Trey could see the blood. Henry had managed to pull out one of his needles and there was blood everywhere. When I say everywhere, that's only a slight exaggeration. He was covered in blood. His shirt, his hands, his bedspread, and especially his sheets, were soaked. It was later the next day when it dawned on me what Henry meant when he said, "I think I wet the bed." That warm, wet fluid wasn't urine. It was blood.

Now I grew up in a family that hunted so I have been around a fair share of grisly, bloody scenes. I'm not grossed out by blood. But what I saw as I started to survey the scene shocked me. The needle he had pulled is the pressurized one used to return the blood into the body. It looked a bit like someone took a garden house of blood and started spraying it around the unit. Henry managed to shoot blood all the way over to my bed about five feet away. In my hundreds of dialysis treatments this was the first time I had someone else's blood on me.

Trey called for Heather, the RN, to assist him as it was apparent that this was a serious situation. Losing so much blood caused Henry's blood pressure to drop like a safe falling off a cliff. I recall Trey saying his pressure was 60/30 at one point. He was fading in and out of consciousness as Trey kept saying, "Henry. Stay with me buddy. Talk to me Henry." He still had one needle in his arm so they started to run fluids into him as fast as they could in an attempt to bring up his BP. Henry rallied a little; enough to tell Trey that he had a "do not resuscitate" order. I remember thinking, "I wonder if he actually does have a DNR or could he just be saying that?" Henry had told me on a couple of different occasions that he was "ready to go" which is a sentiment shared by a lot of dialysis patients. When you're on dialysis, the thought of death certainly isn't terrifying. We're already a little dead anyway.

Of course just because Henry is having a medical emergency doesn't mean other patients will have the common decency not to have problems at the exact same time. After all, there are only two medical personnel and there are ten patients. And sure enough, one of the patients on the other side of the unit needed attention so Heather went to her assistance.

Things went from bad to worse when Trey tried to give Henry a drink of water. I'm not sure why he did that. There was a giant needle in his arm so any fluids that needed to be administered could be pumped directly into his veins. Henry was in bed in an almost completely horizontal position. Trying to give a drink to a very sick man who is flat on his back in bed can easily go wrong and it did. Henry immediately gagged on the water and completely stopped breathing. When water hits the back of the throat there is a survival mechanism that kicks in to keep you from drowning. The throat closes up tight to keep water from going directly into the lungs. Of course, that also makes breathing temporarily impossible. Henry couldn't breathe and started to make violent, panicked movements. His hands shook wildly. Henry's chest and abdomen moved up and down rapidly in no discernable pattern. At that moment, I was sure he was dying and, for some reason, that terrified me. Henry is an old man clinging to life through the help of machines. He is "ready to go" as he told me, and I do not doubt him. His death would not be a tragedy nor would it be unexpected but somehow dying covered in his own blood in a dialysis unit just seemed like a horrible way to go. I had been praying for Henry off and on throughout this whole ordeal but now I started to pray with a newfound sense of purpose. "God, please help Henry. Don't let him die here. His wife will be showing up in a few hours expecting to take him home. Don't let him die like this."

Trey and Heather were trying to figure out what to do. Is he going to pull out of this or should they call 911? It was at that point I whispered, "Maybe you should call the doctor." Heather got on the phone with one of the doctors who runs the unit and tried to convey the seriousness of the situation. The doctor's recommendation was to start the dialysis machine again and get Henry the cleansing he needed. Obviously the seriousness of the situation was lost on him but that's not surprising. He wasn't on the scene. Plus, he seems to be primarily concerned with just keeping us alive. Quality of life? Are you kidding? We're dialysis patients. We don't have a quality of life. Heather and Trey quickly dismissed the idea of restarting dialysis for Henry and called 911. By the time the EMTs arrived Henry had rallied a little and was stabilized.

Once Henry was in the ambulance and on the way to the hospital everyone gave a collective sigh of relief. Trey and Heather then started the unenviable task of cleaning up the blood. When I left at around 4:30 a.m. they were still at it. The smell of bleach burned my nose for those last two hours of treatment. I couldn't have cared less. The ER was nice enough to call down around 4 a.m. and tell Heather that Henry was going to be fine. Obviously he had lost a lot of blood but he was resting comfortably with his wife by his side.

A couple of nights later when I showed up at dialysis Henry was there in his familiar spot. I told him how glad I was to see him and how scared I was that night. He apologized about five times for spraying me with blood. I told him it was no big deal and that I was just very relieved he was okay. What's a little blood between dialysis patients? There was one difference about this night. Both of his hands were restrained. It seemed somewhat cruel but Henry was the one who requested it. I am happy to report that for the rest of the night Henry was as quiet as a church mouse. Let's keep it that way, big fella!

A LUMP

Anyone who as ever tangled with cancer can tell you, it makes you more than a little paranoid. It plants a seed in the back of your mind that probably never gets yanked out all the way to the roots. You are forever changed and find yourself checking things that would never have been noticed prior to your malignancy. "What's that? Shouldn't that be healed by now? Is that a lump? Why does that hurt? Should I mention this to the docs?" I sincerely hope that in time these tendencies go away but somehow I doubt it.

In a weird way, I feel like my body has betrayed me. I know that is completely irrational but that's how I feel. "How could you let that cancer get a hold of you? After all the good things I have done for you over the years. All the exercise, not smoking…have you forgotten I've run almost 1,000 miles a year for the past 25 years. And this is the thanks I get."

The body politely clears its throat and says, "You have got to be kidding me. I notice you didn't mention your diet. You seemed to think that macaroni is a vegetable. And think back to college. It's amazing you still have a liver." The body does have a good memory.

In a way I guess I am lucky given the fact that my type of cancer (clear cell carcinoma) is not known to be aggressive. The doctors are not worried about it spreading. Of course they did every type of scan known to mankind but they really didn't seem concerned that this cancer will spread to the surrounding organs. Still, none of that was running through my head when I discover a lump in my chest. Actually I didn't discover it as much as our dog, Myrna, found it for me. She jumped up putting her paw on my chest and I immediately felt a sharp pain directly below my left nipple. I touched that area and sure enough, there was a lump roughly the size of a quarter. So…shit.

My first thought was, "Ah, it's just a bruise or something. Nothing to worry about. I'll just keep an eye on it and it will probably go away in a week or so." Well, a week came and went and it was still there. If anything, it might even hurt more. I was due to see several doctors on the transplant team in a few days so I decided to bring it up with them. If this was a problem then the best course of action was to deal with it. Ignoring it won't make it go away.

I saw my nephrologist, Dr. Taber, and asked him about the lump. He promptly felt the thing and said, "Yes, that's a lump alright. Sometimes medications can cause those things but not the medications you are on. You ought to get that taken care of." By "taken care of" I knew he meant "cut out." Doctors are nothing if not predictable in that sense and I totally understand. It's a simple decision making process actually. *There's something growing in his body that seems abnormal. Cut it out. End of problem.* That was fine with me. I'm growing accustomed to lidocaine anyway.

I went home and made an appointment with my local doctor but it seemed like I hadn't been able to get in to see him for so long that I wondered if he's still actually my doctor. As usual, I saw a physician's assistant who wasn't nearly as hasty for the knife as I had hoped. I wanted this thing out of me as soon as possible. I felt like saying, "Let me have some lidocaine and I'll do it myself." She wanted me to go for a scan at the local hospital. At first I was frustrated because really, I just wanted this thing cut out of me. I thought, "Well, this thing has *got* to come out. Let's just cut to the chase and schedule the procedure." I went home and did something I should never, ever do. I lied to my wife.

I could not bear the thought of having to tell her I had a lump in my chest. No matter what, I wanted to somehow spare her that worry. Polly is a worrier. She doesn't need any help finding things to worry about. In retrospect, it was a stupid plan. I wasn't sure how I was going to pull this off.

She probably would have noticed the bandages and stitches in my chest. Let me just say I hadn't gotten to that part of my brilliant plan yet. I lied and told Polly I had to go in to work. The rest of my genius plan would come to me later.

A few days later and I was back at Reid Hospital for a scan of my chest. The original plan was to get a scan but when I arrived at Reid I realized I was actually going to have…wait for it…a mammogram. Yes, I was going to have a mammogram which I found odd but then again, what do I know? That's why they let the doctors make the medical decisions. After a few minutes I sort of warmed up to the idea. For years I'd heard women complain about mammograms. Now I was going to get to find out what all the drama was about.

Then, all of a sudden, it got fun. The technician in charge of the mammogram had a preconceived notion that since I was a dude, I would be bothered by having a test that is traditionally given almost exclusively to women. She was worried about damaging my fragile self-image. I thought it was sweet but she couldn't have been more wrong. It was nice of her to go to great lengths to explain that they do give mammograms to men. She said, "Just two weeks ago I gave a mammogram to a man about your age." I tried to explain, "I'm a dialysis patient. Any shred of human dignity I had is long gone. Don't worry about it. It would literally be impossible for you to make me feel shy or embarrassed. Let's just do the test."

She positioned my body up to the machine which was a delicate procedure because, let's face it, I was not well endowed in the breast department. All the female readers know exactly how this test works so this description is strictly for the men. The machine had two clear hard plastic plates that were used to press your breast tissue together. After a couple of minutes of tweaking, the technician had my left breast exactly where she wanted it. I looked down and saw what had to be the funniest sight these eyes have ever seen. My left "man boob" was flattened out and looked very much like a pasty white tostada. I swear that at that moment it was the funniest thing I had ever seen. I started laughing and could not contain myself. I laughed so much they had to wait for me to calm down to do the scan. The technician had to ask me, "Mr. Wilde, please try to hold still." I suddenly had a great idea.

I asked the tech, "Do you happen to have a camera?"

"I'm afraid I don't," she answered.

"A cell phone with a camera. Anything?" I begged.

"No, I'm sorry," she said.

"Would anyone on the floor have a camera?" I asked trying frantically to find a way to preserve this image of my man boob crushed between two sheets of clear plastic. But alas, it was not to be. I missed the opportunity of a lifetime that day. If I had been able to capture that image it would have been my Facebook profile picture forever.

She finished up with the pictures and I got dressed. They took me to a small waiting room and told me they were going to have one of the doctors look at the pictures that day. I was pleasantly surprised because I assumed I'd have to wait several days to get the results. So I waited and waited until the doctor appeared and apologized for the delay. He wasted no time in getting right to the point.

"Mr. Wilde, from looking at your scan and reading over your description that upon the initial onset the lump was painful I am fairly certain I know what we are dealing with here," said the doctor. I almost asked, "So when do we schedule the surgery."

He continued, "What we have here is breast tissue. I'm fairly certain that's all this is. Of course, in medicine you can never be 100% certain but from everything I've looked at I'm confident this is the development of breast tissue, a condition known as gynecomastia."

I was happy that I wouldn't be going under the knife again. I also found a genuine sense of joy at the thought that somehow, at the age of 48, I was developing breasts. Check that, I should have said "breast" as this was only on the left.

"So I'm growing a boob," I asked.

"That's one way to say it I guess," the doctor replied and I could tell he didn't find this nearly as funny as I did. I'm not sure why I thought this was so hysterical. I guess it was the thought, "I'm growing a breast. What's next? When should I expect my vagina to start?"

I asked the doctor, "Do you have any idea why this is happening now?"

"Have you changed or added any medicine recently?" he asked.

"Yes, actually I have. I added a blood pressure medicine about three weeks ago," I answered.

"More than likely, that's the cause," he said as he excused himself to go see another patient who was waiting in another small room. I could only hope that whatever news he delivered to that patient was met with the same joyous enthusiasm. Somehow I doubt it.

As expected, my wife was overjoyed with the news. Well, she wasn't overjoyed that I was growing a breast but she was happy that I didn't have anything more serious to contend with. I apologized for the 500th time for lying to her and swore I'd never, ever do it again. She explained to me that if I ever did lie to her again, my slow transformation into a woman would get sped up dramatically because she would reach down my pants and rip something off to finish the job.

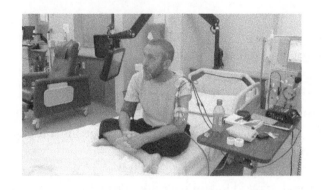

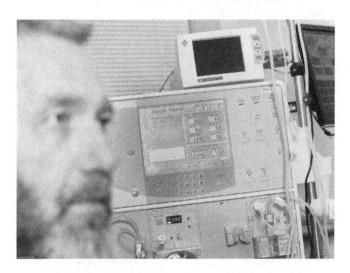

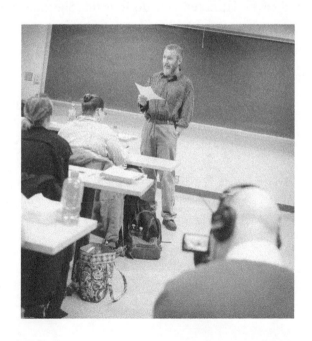

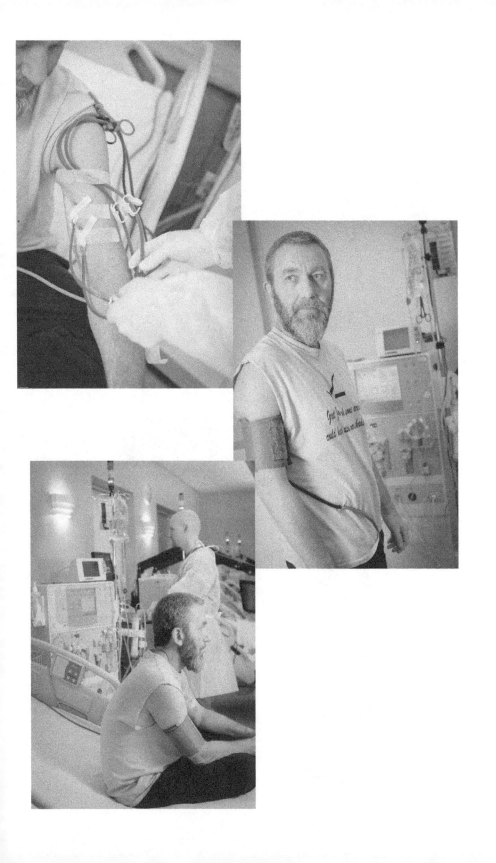

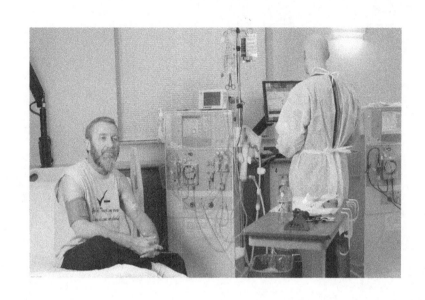

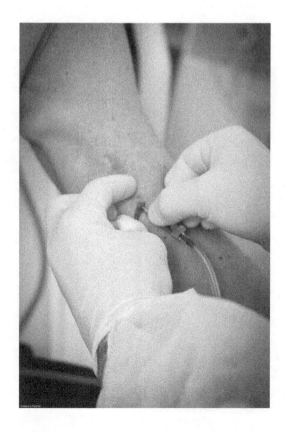

DINNER WITH CURT

When news of my ordeal spread throughout the students at IU East, I was touched by the response. Lots of students stopped by to say "hi" and let me know they were thinking about me. Anyone who has ever been seriously ill will tell you that it means a lot to know people are pulling for you. People feel helpless because there's nothing they can really do but a kind word or a note in the mail means a lot.

There's another group of people who avoid contact because the thought that a friend is sick means, by extension, they could become sick and that scares the shit out of them. I understand that too. The thought of dying is terrifying to most and despite all my bluster about "dialysis patients aren't afraid to die," I'm none too fond of the thought myself. It's not so much the idea of dying that troubles me as the thought of this life being over. Even though I'm sick, life still kicks all kinds of ass. But I am most worried about my family and, more specifically, my kids. My wife is strong. Polly is a rock and eventually she'd be able to put her life back together. That sounds so flippant but it is not intended that way. I know she'd be absolutely devastated but in time, she'd heal. But what about Jawbone Jack and Anna Banana? They are in the throes of adolescence and I think they might need both their parents now more than ever. These years, even more so than childhood, determine what type of person you become. Plus, if I were dead we'd just miss each other so damn much. We have so much fun together.

One of my students who stopped by immediately after hearing I was ill was Curt Deckard. He was one of our nontraditional students who came back to school after exploring other career opportunities. We have a program for adults who have already earned a bachelor's degree and want to become certified to teach. At first I was not a big fan of this type of program because I thought it would bring back the burn-outs who hated their jobs and thought that teaching seemed like an easy gig. I'm happy to say I was wrong. Sure we've had nibbles from lots of slackers over the years but the students who end up in our classrooms are engaged, intelligent, and highly motivated. Virtually every one of these students talks about being "called" to teach and that is exactly what it is…a calling. It's in your bones. Curt had that fire in him, which is how he ended up in my educational psychology class.

Curt is one of those people who, when you meet him, seems like you've known him for years. Some people call these folks "old souls" and that might be a good description. Maybe we did know each other a very long time ago. It almost seems that way sometimes. Curt used to sit in the far back corner of my class and continuously crack up everyone in the room…me included. Several times I would be laughing so hard at one of his one-liners that I would have to turn around and face the chalkboard until I could put on a serious professor face. Most times I just went with the moment and laughed along with everyone else. I unofficially became Curt's mentor and he would seek me out when he had an issue or just needed some advice. He's a great guy and I was sad when he graduated. I was happy for him but sad that we wouldn't be seeing each other all that often anymore.

The summer after his graduation he emailed me a few times asking when I would be in my office. It was during the part of the summer when I wasn't working on campus so I'd always write back, "I'm not really going to be on campus for awhile." I assumed he just wanted to get together and shoot the breeze. After a few emails back and forth he asked if Polly and I wanted to join him and his wife for dinner. That seemed like a great idea. He also mentioned that he wanted to talk to me about something. I assumed it was job related as he had just earned his license and was in the middle of job hunting.

We met later that week on Friday night at Chili's after running the kids around to band and baseball practice. We engaged in the typical small talk

for awhile (i.e., "How's the summer going?" "How are the kids?") until Curt
said, "I suppose you are wondering why I asked you here?" Actually, I was
wondering but I thought it was just a chance to get together and, like I said,
maybe talk about strategies for landing him that first job. He said, "Stephanie
and I have talked about this and we'd like to know if you'd be interested in
me giving you one of my kidneys." Excuse me? Could you say that again?
You'd like to give me one of your kidneys! Holy smokes! I accept.

Needless to say, I was stunned. I stammered something like, "Well, that
would be great but have you really thought this through?" And here's where
the story gets even better. As it turns out Curt *had* thought this out. He's been
thinking it out for a long time. His father had received a heart transplant 21
years ago and has been doing great ever since. His father's first heart attack
was when Curt was quite young and his Dad made nearly a full recovery.
However, his father suffered a second, much more damaging heart attack,
when Curt was in his early teens and the effects were much more pervasive.
Curt said that everything about their family changed after this second heart
attack. Everything had to be considered in the light of his father's health.
I got it. I knew exactly what he meant because that is the way our family
is when I'm sick. Every decision has to be run through the "Dad-o-meter"
before reaching a conclusion. Is Dad strong enough? Will it conflict with his
dialysis schedule?

Curt's father was at death's door. The doctors at Ball Memorial Hospital
in Muncie, Indiana gave him 72 hours to live. They told Curt's mother that
she should start planning his funeral. That seemed like as good a time as any
to look for a new hospital and thank God they did. He was transferred to
Methodist in Indianapolis with literally hours to live. In those final hours a
match was found and he was given the most fantastic gift ever imagined…a
brand spanking new lease on life. You see, it not just that you get to live
longer. You get to live longer and it feels like you are in the body of a
15-year-old. The Deckard family has now received 21 extra years with their
patriarch. That's 21 years of the good shit. The graduations, the marriages,
the grandchildren…the peak of the mountain shit that would have been just

a little hollow without "dad" and "grandpa" there. Now there is not a need to say, "Dad would have loved this." He *is* loving this. Look at him!

That's what Curt wants to give to me. He wants to make sure I get to see the day my beautiful daughter finds a man good enough to be her husband. Curt wants to make sure I am there to make sure I approve of this guy (yeah, right...like there's a guy on this planet deserving of my Anna.) He wants me to walk her down the aisle. Curt probably knows that my boy needs more work on his curveball. His breaking ball is good for a 12-year-old but he needs constant reminders to bend his back and stay on top of the ball. Curt wants to make sure that I'm there when Jack makes batters look ridiculous chasing his curveball. Curt wants Polly and me to grow old together. He wants us to have those quiet evenings on the back deck with a bottle of wine and a fire to keep away the chill. He wants us to spoil our grandchildren rotten. He wants us to feed those grandkids ice cream for breakfast, which is a tradition in my family. Curt wants that so much that he's willing to go into a hospital and give a part of himself to make sure my family has all that and more. He did have some strings though. He wanted a guaranteed "A" in any graduate course I taught and he said he didn't really even want to do the work. That's it? For that I get a kidney? Deal!

He asked me at dinner, "What blood type are you?"

"I'm A positive."

He smiled, "Me too."

"Well, that's a good first step but they still have to do much more testing to determine if we're a match," I acknowledged.

It gets even weirder. It turns out that one of his very best friends in high school is the head of organ procurement at University Hospitals where I am being treated. She already talked to her and she answered most of his questions. He was ready to go. If one of the surgeons would have said we could do the surgery that night Curt would have jumped up on the operating table.

Flash forward a few months. Curt has to lose eleven more pounds before they will do the testing to see if we are a match. He's been trying hard but has been struggling with a painful case of plantar fasciitis. It's hard to be very active when your feet hurt like hell with each step. So we wait but I've got plenty of time. Just the thought that someone would go through all the pain of an operation just for me is mind-boggling. I'm certain I don't deserve that kind of sacrifice but you can be certain I'm going to do everything I can to make myself worthy even if it is after the fact.

I HATE CHRISTIAN ROCK

We have a massive deck on the back of our house. We love to roast marshmallows in the fire pit and grill out during the summer. It ruined our kickball field in the backyard but it was worth it. Of course there is a down side to the deck. To make sure it doesn't decay from rain and weather, each summer I slather on a coat of Thompson's Water Seal. Before the slathering begins, I have to clean all the dirt off the deck, which is quite an undertaking but something that absolutely needs to be done. We paid a small fortune for this damn deck. I could have bought a nice used car with what we paid for the deck so it gets good care each summer.

On day three of the slathering process, I started to feel rather poorly. I was tired but then again, I am always tired. "I should be tired from all this work," I thought to myself as I dabbed on the final touches of the second coat of water seal. Sleep took me right about the time my head hit the pillow later that afternoon. My wife came up to check on me after a few hours and said, "You feel hot. You're burning up." I told her it was hot out on the deck when I was doing all that slathering. She said, "That was four hours ago. You shouldn't still feel this hot," as she went to get the thermometer. The verdict was 103 degrees. So...shit.

Polly called the dialysis center and they recommended a trip to the ER. A fever is a sign that I could have an infection in my catheter. My brother's words were ringing in my head. "It's not a question of 'if' it'll get infected. It's a question of 'when' it'll get infected." So off to the ER I went.

At the intake station they took my temperature and much to my surprise, it had dropped. It was almost in the normal range. For just a second I thought about saying, "Well, I guess that was a false alarm" and heading home. I knew if I did that Polly would put her size 7 shoe right up my butt and make me go back so I stayed. They took me back to my own private little area with a TV and everything. This was by far the nicest ER I've ever been to and I've been to a few. I've been to restaurants that weren't this nice.

As you might expect, I waited quite a while. Eventually a doctor came in and explained that the real danger was an infection in my catheter. If there was an infection, it could spread into my blood and turn into sepsis which could mean "game over." They were going to take blood from my arm to check for infection in my system and also from my catheter to see if that was infected. They harpooned my arm and drew a sample which was sent to the lab. Then it got tricky. They had to draw blood from my catheter. It seems that there is a universal understanding that unless you are a dialysis nurse, you never, ever mess with a catheter. It's a bad idea to even say "catheter." The mere mention of the word triggers a pre-programmed response, "We're told never to do anything with catheters." But now the team in the ER had no choice. They had to draw blood from a catheter so they literally went to the procedural manual to get the instructions for this rarest of rare procedures. None of the ER nurses had ever done it before.

A team of about a half dozen nurses and techs were in my room for the draw. One had the job of reading the instructions while another performed the procedure. The reader went line by line down the procedural manual and often had to reread certain directions. "Release the clamp."

"So should I do that now?" said the nurse working on my catheter.

"That's what it says," responded the nurse with the directions.

Eventually they drew my blood and I got to go home and wait for the lab results. Meanwhile, I was told to fight the fever with Tylenol which actually worked quite well. The next time I went to dialysis my temperature was gone. I assumed I had caught a bug somewhere and all the blood draws were "much ado about nothing." While I was sitting in my chair watching the clock and wishing I had the mental powers to control the flow of time, a nurse came over and said, "The results from the lab came back and your catheter is infected. The good news is they found no sign of infection in your blood."

"So what does that mean?" I asked.

"You have to have your catheter replaced," she said. "We've already made an appointment for you. It's the day after tomorrow."

"Shit." I thought. It's always something. Never ends.

I wasn't too worried about having my catheter replaced because putting it in was no big deal. Switching it out for a new one would probably be about the same I assumed. *Big mistake!* You all know the expression, "Never assuming anything because there are different protocols for different surgical procedures." That's an oldie but it's so true. I assumed I'd be consciously sedated like last time. Nope. What they can do is give you a Xanax five minutes prior to the procedure that will do nothing to help with the pain but at least you'll be a little more relaxed.

So they wheel me into the room and there is music playing. However, it is not AC/DC like last time. I am a huge fan of rock music and listen to most of the different genres and subgenres but this is foreign to me. How could that be? I am puzzled for a moment and then the lyrics gave me a clue. This is Christian rock.

While I am a Christian, I absolutely loathe Christian rock. Rock-n-roll is about rebellion. It's music that should piss off your parents, no matter how old. It should make you want to give the middle finger to any and all authority figures. Christian rock is defiling that ethos. It's combining rebellious, anti-establishment music with lyrics about Jesus and when He will return. While Jesus was as revolutionary as any man in history, the practice of organized religion is not exactly radical by any stretch of the imagination. Organized religion can be incredibly boring and mundane; something rock should never be. Christian rock is like peanut butter and mustard. On their own, they are both delicious but they should never be eaten together.

So they coated me in freezing cold betadine and the fun started. The doctor told me that she was going to start injecting the lidocaine and that I'd feel a little sting. I've had lidocaine plenty of times and it's not that big a deal. However, this time it was really hurting and I'm not sure why. It was probably because I was not expecting this procedure to be painful. I've had a lot of painful medical procedures so I am not a wussy when it comes to pain. I can man up and take it when I need to. But this procedure was starting to kick my ass. The doc then did what had to be done. She started yanking my infect catheter out of me. That hurt. I mean that really hurt. The lidocaine was just numbing my skin and did nothing for the deeper tissue. I was biting down on my lip and trying to take it in silence. "A few more yanks and it'll all be over," I told myself. Finally the pain became more than I could contain and I cry out, "Owww…that really hurts. Is it suppose to hurt this much?" I was thinking, "Why couldn't I be sedated a bit? Are they trying to save money and not use the meds?"

More tugs and I'm getting in a bad mood. The pain, the freezing cold betadine, and that music…that awful Christian rock was the final straw. I said, "This is really painful. Why is it hurting this much?"

The doctor said, "Well, we're working in an area that is infected so that doesn't feel good."

"Why aren't you giving me something for the pain?" I asked.

"Well, we usually don't do that when replacing a catheter," was the answer.

Now I was pissed. I'm having a catheter jerked out of my chest and they are playing Christian rock. Christian rock!

I half yell, "And that music is NOT helping either."

Looks of bewilderment surround me, "Do you want it turned off?" someone asks.

"I don't care now. It's just that I HATE CHRISTIAN ROCK," I practically scream.

The looks on the faces that surround me were ones of, "Do we have a psycho on our hands?" I realized I was not being a "good patient" so I shut up. They wouldn't understand anyway. No, I'm not a psycho. I'm a dialysis patient and I'm sick of being poked and prodded. I'm sick of surgical theatres and dialysis. I sick of my body. I'm sick of people seeing me and saying, "You look great." I'm sick of this life. And dear God, I despise Christian rock. Go ahead and worship the Lord but please do not attempt to "rock out." You look like a friggin' idiot.

I regained my composure at that point and they finished the procedure, taped me up, and sent me home. Of course I had dialysis that night so they could test out my new catheter. It worked great so at least it was inserted correctly. Side note: I was scheduled to have another surgery to try and create a fistula again but that is going to have to wait for a few weeks now until they run me through a course of antibiotics. Wow! That was an ordeal I could have done without.

FOR IT IS BY GRACE
YOU HAVE BEEN SAVED

Curt Deckard and his family stopped over last night. It was an unannounced visit and they came bearing a gift. They had a two-liter jug of Diet Mt. Dew (also known around the Wildehouse as "nectar of the gods") wrapped in a gift bag. I had a habit of always drinking Diet Mt. Dew during class. Actually I had a habit of drinking Diet Mt. Dew unless I was asleep. Curt told me, "Well, I know you can't have this now but in a few months you'll be able to again. We're a match." I had just finished running on the treadmill so I was dripping with sweat and smelly but I gave him a big hug anyway.

We invited Curt and his family in to bask in the complete awesomeness of the moment. I already had met Stephanie, his wife, on a few occasions but now I was able to see his children, Elizabeth and T.C. At one point I asked his children how they felt about their Dad donating a kidney to me. T.C. spoke up and said, "Nervous."

I said, "I understand that. You love your Dad and want to make sure he's okay. You probably feel a lot like my kids feel when I'm having some kind of surgery."

Our daughter looked at me and said, "You always say, 'it's no big deal, don't worry' but I do." And then Curt said something that made everything click into place for me. You see, I was having a hard time understanding why someone would make such a tremendous sacrifice for me. He was a student of mine sure, but trust me, I'm not that great of an instructor that students offer up their organs every semester. As it turned out, when this ordeal was taking place, he was student teaching in Anna's high school. On the days following my surgery, Curt said he could look at Anna and see the worry on her face. Even though she was trying to be brave, he said he could see it on her. He said, "And that was me when I was about her age." He recognized that frightened kid in his class. He recognized himself. And now, as an adult, he could do something to take away that fear. He could save my life. That's when I finally got it. Why would someone go through major surgery to help someone else? First, they have to just be that kind of person. There are not many of them but they are out there. Curt Deckard is living proof. I was extremely fortunate that our paths crossed. Sometimes it's better to be lucky than good. Second, in some way, Curt was trying to do what we'd all like to do. Rewrite the parts of our lives that really, really sucked. He couldn't rewrite his own history but he damn well could change Anna's. He couldn't escape those months and years of worrying about his father. He could, however, ease that burden for one young lady. Oh yeah, and he could also set aside years of dialysis and save my life. That's not too bad either.

Curt still has to have a battery of tests to make certain there is nothing wrong with him medically that would prevent him from donating. This is another step in the journey but let's be clear. It's a freakin' huge step. People use the phrase, "three little words" and for most people, it means, "I love you." For me, those three little words are "we're a match."

PRAISE GOD

It's been an interesting few days. Last Friday (September 17, 2010), the local paper ran an article about Curt and me. The title was "Ex-Student Donating Kidney to Professor." In fact, it was on the front page of the paper with a very nice picture of yours truly smiling at my students. A photographer came to one of my classes and took about 187 pictures and the paper actually printed two (along with a headshot of Curt). Everyone could use a "feel good story" once in awhile, but for me the whole point of the article was to raise awareness of the need for more organ donors. As Curt said, "When people think about organ donation, they usually think you have to die to be a donor. You don't. Almost anyone can be a donor." And, I have to admit, it's a pretty good story.

Since the article came out I've been getting stopped everywhere by people with congratulations and kind words. I've heard from colleagues who said, "I didn't know you were sick." College professors don't get out much, I guess. It's nice to get some attention but trust me when I say, that's not why I agreed to do the article. I was hoping to raise awareness but I also wanted Curt to get some recognition because what he is doing is truly a remarkable act of love, kindness, and generosity. Just for a moment, think about what he is *volunteering* to do. Curt is going to go into a hospital for 3-4 days, be cut open, have a major organ removed, and experience a considerable amount of pain for his trouble. And what does he get out of it? Two things…a really sexy scar and the right to walk around knowing he did something that 99.9%

of people would never have the courage to do. Heck, most people would never even consider it.

And while I am completely blown away by the thought of someone being willing to make that type of sacrifice, that's *not* what I'm thinking about tonight. In fact, it's 2:30 a.m. and I finally decided to get up and head down to the computer. Maybe writing about this will help me wrap my head around it and I'll be able to get some sleep.

A student stopped in my office today. She saw the article and wanted to congratulate me. I explained that Curt was going to donate a kidney and we had recently learned we are a match. She said, "Praise God. He works miracles every day." We continued chatting about my health concerns and, as it turned out, she had some health problems of her own. In our conversation she repeatedly kept coming back to "Praise God." For some reason, I was getting annoyed with that and finally said, "Well, you know, God could have spared everyone a lot of trouble and just not given me cancer." I think that went completely over her head or she thought I was joking.

Like a lot of people, she had cast her gaze upon the Lord and, despite my efforts to have her consider another possibility, she couldn't seem to look away. Instead of praising God, how about praising Curt? Isn't he the one making this possible? How about praising the doctors for dedicating their lives to medicine and making organ donation a possibility? How about praising my wife for taking care of my sick ass for all these years? She never complains and I know how worried she is about me. I'd do anything to take that worry away but singlehandedly, Curt is taking care of that for me.

If God deserves the credit for this miracle, then doesn't He deserve some of the blame, too? God could have stepped in at almost any juncture and made Curt's heroics completely unnecessary. The Almighty could have given me a good pair of kidneys to start with rather than letting Alport Syndrome have its way with me. He could have made the tumor on my transplanted kidney benign. Heck, he could have zapped the tumor when it was tiny. I know some people would say that God is directing Curt to help me. Maybe He is talking to Curt. But Curt still has got to be willing to listen. Most of us are pretty good at turning a deaf ear to the suffering of others. I know I am. I get too wrapped up in my own issues to pay attention.

And, who knows, maybe this is all part of God's plan for me. Maybe all this pain and suffering is for a good reason. When Curt stopped over to our house a few weeks ago with the news that we were a match, I thanked God. I told our kids, "We are definitely going to church this Sunday. We've got so much to be grateful for." But there is also a part of me that is pissed off because I have to endure all this. I try not to say, "Why me? What have I done to deserve this?" because I know there is no answer to that question. At least there's no answer that's going to satisfy me so I try not to think about it. It just seems that if people are willing to give God all the credit, then He deserves some of the blame too. I'm sure He can handle it. He's God.

Maybe we could share some of the miracle making with Curt. He's *living* the Golden Rule. He's putting himself at risk to help his fellow man. He's making an incredible sacrifice for me. Curt is giving me a second chance at life. That sure sounds praise-worthy to me.

THE ART AND SCIENCE
OF SCRATCHING

As you know by now, my skin itches. I will not waste any more ink reiterating how bothersome my itching has become but suffice to say it is driving me crazier than a shithouse mouse. My skin itches all the time; literally, all of the time.

Since itchy skin has become a central feature of my life, I thought I'd spend a little time explaining the nuances of scratching. I am, after all, an expert. There are several factors to take into consideration when you go in for a scratch. What follows is the latest research coupled with the personal insights from a master of every stroke from the "sweep and drag" to the "digging for gold."

First, you must consider your instruments. I tend to be old fashioned so my weapons of choice are my hands. I am a maestro with these ten digits. Keep in mind if you're going to go old school like me, you have to be cognizant of fingernail maintenance. What I mean by that is for you to achieve maximum effect, your nails can't be either too long or too short. If they are too short, you are wasting scratching capacity. You need at least $1/4^{th}$ of an inch separation between nails and fingertips. Anything less and the fingertips make contact with the skin and interfere with the "digging of nail on flesh" which is the desired effect. Keep in mind that there are some scratchologists who prefer the "rubbing" of the back. They are in the minority and are largely discredited by the scientific community. Rubbing may occasionally be a nice alternative to the "scorched earth" policy employed by most people but many in the community disavow rubbing altogether as a waste of time that could be used providing relief with a good raking of the flesh. The choice is yours.

I should warn you that excessive nail length can be problematic, too. If your nails are too long you risk the possibility of the dreaded "fold back." The fold back is when you apply excessive pressure and your finger nails actually "fold back" which, in clinical terms, "hurts like hell." Trust me, you don't want that. What we're looking for here is 1/4th of an inch clearance and scratchologists such as me have devised a simple technique to determine if you have proper nail/finger clearance.

You can use a procedure similar to the one used when checking the tread on a tire. To make sure you have sufficient tread on your tire, you place a penny into the tread and if Abe Lincoln's head is still visible, you're in good shape. When making a similar determination of nail length, rather than using a penny, substitute a quarter. Simply put the quarter directly under your fingernail and above the flesh of your finger. If the top of George Washington's noggin in still visible, you have excellent nail/finger tip separation. Now let's get to the scratching.

Pressure is also a factor to consider. It is a personal choice and each scratcher and scratchee must find the proper pressure for maximum relief. Too much and you risk puncturing the skin which can lead to infection in the worst-case scenario and a nasty "mess" in the least. There have been times where I have made myself bleed from applying excessive pressure. Generally this is not a problem but in cases of extreme itch attacks, one generally is in such a state of pain that ripping away layers of skin is quite possible and can actually go unnoticed.

One way to minimize this possibility is to make certain scratching is not taking place too soon after a nail trimming. The danger in trimming is that sharp edges can, and often do, appear. The edges require a radical adjustment of torque. If the previous levels of torque are applied post-trimmage, you're headed for trouble. Ease way back on the torque until you've established that there are no sharp edges. I can think of an instance when my son had recently trimmed his nails and was scratching my back. It felt, in a word, amazing. A few minutes after the session, I was experiencing discomfort. I asked my wife to look at my back and immediately heard a loud gasp. My son had filleted my back. I was cut and bleeding. My back hurt like heck for two days.

Another cautionary tale is when nails are broken or bitten off. There is a higher possibility of the creation of the dreaded "nail-blade." The nail-blade can accidentally cause a considerable amount of damage. For example, I noticed in dialysis that I had a toenail that was growing out of control and simply tore off the edge during treatment. You tend to notice things like that when you are trapped in a bed for six hours at a time. Later in the night I had an itch on my lower calf and used my foot to scratch it. The next morning I noticed the area was sore so I looked to see two horizontal cuts on my leg. The nail-blade had done the damage so please, be careful out there.

It's time to move from the "old school" use of hands and explore the tools that are often employed by professional scratchologists. Obviously the most common is the back scratcher. Several dialysis patients rely heavily on various forms of the back scratcher and I am one of them. There are numerous styles to choose from and I encourage you to try them out before selecting yours. Be cognizant of two factors when making your selection: reach and angle. The scratcher has to be long enough to reach all offending appendages. Angle is more of a personal choice which is why it is important to try them out before making a choice. Remember that variety is the spice of life so change your angle every 3-5 seconds.

Many scratchers enjoy plying their trade in more of an improvisational manner. They are comfortable using any and all surfaces as potential sources of relief. I encourage each and every reader to get creative. A few classics should be mentioned however.

Door jambs – always an option as virtually every room in the house has one.

Walls – the old style 1970s paneling is the best.

Household appliances - use the hard edges and/or corners.

Any handheld device – think "spatula."

Most of all, get creative and have fun scratching that itch.

It's time to move on into more detailed discussion of scratching as we turn our attention to various positions one must strike in order to get maximum relief. The following section largely applies to scratching while in a bed but could also be applicable if you find yourself in a barcalounger or recliner.

The scratching lotus – a position that requires a well-conditioned set of abdominal muscles. The first step is to extend your legs and arch your back. This will allow you to achieve "ass-clearance" as, if you are doing the scratching lotus correctly, your butt will now elevate above the chair or bed. The next step is to get in there quickly and scratch where it itches while remaining aware of the fact that your stomach muscles are not what they used to be and could give out at any second. Speed is of the essence. Get in there and get the job done.

The itchy dragon – a variation of the scratching lotus for those who cannot achieve ass elevation. The itchy dragon starts by swinging one leg across the other. This will allow you to attack the area that needs relief. Feel free to be a switch hitter and alternate between left and right cheek with the itchy dragon.

The rubbing giraffe – is a rarely used technique typically only needed when the scratcher has some impediment using his/her arm(s). For example, if he/she had two enormous needles stuck in an arm and had to keep said arm still or said needles will become dislodged creating what is known as the "blood super soaker." The rubbing giraffe can generally be thought of as any technique where the head is used as a scratching tool. For example, using ones noggin to scratch an arm would be considered the rubbing giraffe. Rubbing is used here because technically, the head contains no sharp edges, only mildly abrasive surfaces like an eyebrow or a beard.

The chafing cheetah – is generally thought of as any technique employed in a full-on itch attack. The key here is speed, frenzy, and creativity. If scratching were musicianship, think of the chafing cheetah as an all-star jam session. Anything and everything is allowed and even encouraged. Kitchen utensils? Sure! TV remote controls? Absolutely! Having your dog hop up on you and then switch him around so his claws are digging into your back? Not a problem. The only limitations with the chafing cheetah are in your mind.

I sincerely hope you leave this chapter better informed about the art and science of scratching. Remember the keys: instrument of choice, nails, torque, trimmage, tools, and positions. INTTTP is a useful mnemonic or some prefer the key word technique of "I Need To Totally Take a Pee" which of course is easy for a dialysis patient to remember since we never do. Good luck and happy scratching!

THE BURDEN

Things have gone from strange to stranger here at Camp Dialysis. After an incredible emotional high when we found out that Curt was a match, we were all bummed out by the news that his second set of labs was not good. In fact, he was in the "pre-diabetic" range which is certainly problematic if you are hoping to be a donor and should be down-right scary for anyone under any circumstances. Diabetes is no joke. I didn't understand what a horrible disease it was until I was on dialysis. Diabetics are a common sight in dialysis centers. In 2005, diabetes was the primary cause of kidney failure in 43% of dialysis patients. Diabetics have a twelve times greater chance of having end stage renal failure than non-diabetics. Kidney failure is just one of the many problems associated with diabetes. Maybe it's a blessing in disguise that Curt found out now.

So the first concern was for Curt's long-term health. Maybe this will serve as a wake-up call and he will make some healthier life choices. Things like this explain why people who chose to be donors actually have a slightly longer life expectancy than the general population. Curt explained that the docs thought his pre-diabetic reading may be simply a matter of him needing to lose weight. So he's got to lose weight before they'll re-do the labs. If the results of his labs are good then he'll have to continue to lose weight before he's eligible to donate. So…shit.

I get the feeling more and more each day that I am running out of time. The longer I'm on dialysis, the sicker I get. My labs are still atrocious even though I'm doing six hours of dialysis. I'm chronically sleep-deprived, skinny, and just plain sick. The last time I was on dialysis I developed new symptoms every few months. Like all of a sudden all the hair on my arms and legs fell out. Weird. Then my feet gradually lost feeling until they were constantly numb. I'm not exactly sure what causes things like that but I think it's just the impact of having all those toxins swimming around in me for so long. Those toxins caused nerve damage from the inside out, which eventually caused the numbness. Maybe I won't have those symptoms this time or maybe I just haven't been on dialysis long enough to get there. There's just more and more stuff going wrong in my body and I can't help but think… tick-tock, tick-tock.

And let me just get this out: the next person who says, "You look good," is going to get slapped. I don't care who it is. If a nine-year-old tells me I look good, he's going down! I never know what to say to that. I used to say, "Yeah, I'm hanging in there," but lately I've started saying, "I'm not dead yet" which makes folks uncomfortable. I wonder how many people look at me and think, "What are his diet secrets?" My diet secrets? *Cancer,* baby. *Dialysis,* sweetheart. You should try it. The weight just falls off.

This illness is a burden and it gets heavier with each passing day. I've said time and time again that you can't get too up or too down on this journey. I made a mistake when I found out Curt was a match. I started envisioning an end to this misery. I saw myself hunched over a bowl of ice cream, getting a great night's sleep again, and making love to my wife like we were bunnies. Let me clarify…those were separate fantasies, not concurrent. Even though I was saying all the right things such as, "There's still a lot of things that have to happen before this transplant can take place," in my head I was thinking about the other side. I was thinking about laying this burden down. Big mistake. I may be ready to be done with dialysis but dialysis isn't done with me.

So now what? I have to readjust my expectations and accept the fact that there is a lot more dialysis in my future. I don't know what I can do to help Curt. I've offered to do anything. I told him I work out every day. It would be easy enough to drive up to his place and work out with him. My guess is he'd like to handle this privately and I can certainly understand that.

I'm trying to play mental games to make things easier. Surely that is the sign of a desperate man. Lately I've been trying to learn to love the needles. After all, it is the needles that bring me life. Sure they hurt a little but that pain is the price I pay for additional time on this earth. I can take it. Right now there's only one way out and I still plan on sticking around for a while. I tell myself, "The needles are my friends. They are giving me life." I keep saying that and it might be working. But, for the love of God, hurry up Curt. I'm not sure how long I can hang on.

SEX ON DIALYSIS

For those of you waiting for a lurid tale of sexual adventures taking place at a dialysis center near you, sorry, but that's not what this chapter is about. Although I have to confess I have no idea what the staff does when things are quiet in the middle of the night. I sincerely doubt any hanky-panky is taking place. I'll keep a closer watch and get back to you on that one.

This entry is about the challenges of trying to have some type of normal sex life while suffering from a life-changing illness. I'm not going to lie, it's been a burden. The biggest trick is finding a time when my penis feels like cooperating. He seems to have developed a mind of his own. When my wife and I are interlocked in an amorous embrace, he's not interested. When it's 3 am and the missus is sound asleep, he's raring to go. What a dick!

And then when schedules do align, he losses interest half way through. My long-suffering wife, Polly, has been great throughout all this. She talks to me the way a baseball coach talks to a hitter in a prolonged slump.

"That's okay. We'll get 'em next time."

"Good effort. All you can do is keep working at it."

"Keep your weight back."

"Stop lunging."

"Those bloopers are bound to drop in eventually."

Okay, that last one only relates to baseball but you get the picture. We had to resort to the kind of sex life I had in high school. I won't give too many details but let's just say I haven't had to open any jars for my wife lately.

These sexual difficulties bother me and the fact that it bothers me, bothers me. I thought I was past all that. I pride myself on *not* being a misogynistic, macho shithead. We've got way too many of those folks already. I saw plenty of them when I was doing couple's therapy. Good Lord the stories I could tell you if it weren't for client-therapist confidentiality.

There's a lot that goes into being a man and 97.5% of it doesn't relate to what occurs in the bedroom. It's about bringing home a paycheck each month and helping with homework. It's about being a good father to your children and really listening to your wife when she needs to talk. Yes, a lot of those silly stereotypes are absolutely true. Polly rarely needs me to solve her problems but she often likes to explain them to me. That helps her work through them and all I really need to do is give her my full, undivided attention.

Being a man isn't about the amount of your salary, the car you drive, or any of that stupid stuff. Then why are these sexual problems bothering me? I know that once I get a new kidney my wife is going to be in *real* trouble. I keep telling her that too. "When I get a kidney, you and me, baby! Just you wait." These troubles are because I am really sick. I get that.

It could be my real concern is really for my wife. She likes sex, too. Maybe my worries aren't generated from my ego as much as it is from a deep concern about her happiness. That seems plausible. Nah…someone needs to call "bullshit" on me because I'm too much of a selfish jerk for that to be the primary cause. I'm not saying that isn't part of it but that's not the whole reason. Maybe it's because there's more misogynistic shit-headedness in me than I'd care to admit. That fits a whole lot better. Oh well…I'm still willing to empty the dishwasher and that's got to count for something.

THE SIX THINGS I WILL
MISS WHEN I'M DEAD

I've been thinking more and more about death these past few months. I waffle between being optimistic about the possibility of surviving long enough to get a transplant and then assessing my chances realistically and thinking, "doubtful." Some people manage dialysis better than others. I used to be on a shift with a guy who had been on dialysis for fourteen years. Of course, he looks terrible but he's still among the living. I wouldn't bet a plug nickel I could last another fourteen months, let alone fourteen years.

My life is winding down. That is true regardless of the status of my transplant. This would seem to be a good time to reflect on the things I will miss the most when I'm gone. A little thought and reflection may provide the opportunity to learn something before I go belly up.

I sincerely hope there is a place called heaven and that I've lived my life in a way that would get this poor soul inside. But the truth is I haven't the faintest clue if there's an afterlife and that's fine with me. People who tell you they "know" there is a heaven are probably trying to convince themselves just as much as trying to persuade you. How can anyone "know?" I understand that lots of people "believe" with all their hearts but that's not the same as knowing. Maybe people are afraid to answer that still, small voice that comes to each of us in the middle of the night. Maybe they're afraid that if they question the existence of heaven, they will be punished. Would simply questioning and harboring a doubt earn you a one-way ticket to the lake of fire? I sure hope not because I'm probably screwed then but I can't imagine why God would give us these large brains and then say, "But don't use them too much." It makes no sense. If blind allegiance was His goal, then why not make us all simpletons? Problem solved! Knock forty points of most people's IQs and they won't question anything. But still, I can't imagine living my life in fear of some eternal retribution. If that's why people behave themselves, well, that's weak. How about living a good life simply because that's the right thing to do? I try to live in a way that will bring about a better world simply by treating everyone with kindness, respect, and decency. I've never understood why anyone would need anything more than that. But I digress. Thanks for letting me get that off my chest. I feel better. And your prayers for my eternal soul are appreciated.

The things I will miss the most (in no particular order):

1. The smell of barbeque – It's not just the smell that is so intoxicating but what the barbeque symbolizes. Barbeque = summer and summer = fun! More precisely, summer is the season of baseball, long days, sunshine, and summer break.

    But let's get back to our friend the barbeque for a minute because I'm still trying to articulate exactly what it is about the smell of the barbeque that makes me downright giddy. Well, for starters, any food that is barbequed is automatically 26% better tasting than if it were prepared some other way. Someone could grill a tennis ball and if it was covered in just enough sauce, I'd probably take a bite or two. I'm notorious for getting really cheap steaks but after I cook them on the grill, they taste like filet mignon.

    There are other reasons to hail the grill. The smell of the grill always makes me think of the song "Burn, Baby, Burn" by the greatest American band of all time, the Dictators. The Ramones had nothing on these guys. Any band that writes a song about barbequing is okay in my book. Also, any band that has a lead singer who was a former professional wrestler is doing something right. HDM…King of Men!

Grilling out always makes me think of our first dog, Theo. He was an old boy when we rescued him from the pound. It's probably not the best move to adopt a seven-year-old dog but what were we going to do, leave him there? When he lifted his leg and peed through the fence into the other dog's cage, I knew he was the one. Theo used to love it when we grilled out because he would get out afterwards and lick all the grease off the bottom of the grill. When he was working over a grill, he was in dog heaven. Theo didn't just lick our grill. He kept the whole neighborhood clean. So when I smell the grill, I am immediately reminded of Theo, the Dictators, and awful meat. Life is good.

Baseball – I can practically hear people muttering "typical guy" when I bring up baseball but hear me out. My love of the game has a lot more to do with what goes on outside the white lines than the actual game. Okay, that's not completely true. I love the strategy of baseball, too.

When people complain that baseball is boring I know immediately that they don't understand the intricacies of the game. To the uninitiated, baseball is just people throwing a ball back a forth between the pitcher and catcher. Every once in awhile, the batter hits it and all hell breaks loose for a few seconds. That *would* be boring but there's so much more going on that people are missing. There's the cat and mouse game between hitter and pitcher. Let's say there's a man on second and no one out. The hitter's job is to get that runner over to third so someone else can drive him in with either a sacrifice fly, ground out, or base hit. The pitcher knows exactly what the batter is trying to do and his job is to keep that runner at second base. So the pitcher is going to trying to pitch the ball inside to a right-handed batter so it's difficult to hit the ball towards second base. Whichever player is successful in these types of situations largely determines the outcomes of the game. I could write five pages about that scenario alone but I'll spare you.

Real baseball fans are already going over these scenarios in their heads (Who's hitting? Can he bunt? What type of defense alignment should the opposing manager try? Who covers third base? Should the hitter take a strike and try to determine if the third baseman is going to play back or charge? If he takes a strike will they change the defensive alignment?). So, yes, I confess, I love the strategy involved but what I really love is the lessons that can be learned about life through baseball.

I played high school baseball for Gene Schultz who holds the national record for the most wins in a career. Coach Schultz came to a little town in northeastern Iowa when he was fresh out of college and built a baseball dynasty. He has over 1600 wins and numerous state titles. In all of the games I played for Coach Schultz, never once did he mention anything about winning a game. It never came up… not once. We won four state championships but he never discussed winning. We had no gimmicks. Our team had good players but very few, if any, great players. Our focus was on the fundamentals. That was our big secret. We were going to catch the ball and throw it to the correct base. We ran the bases hard which put pressure on the other teams' defenses. Our pitchers didn't walk many batters. Like I said, we played the game the right way and let winning and losing take care of itself. Can you see the lesson here? *Do things the right way.* That's it. Let me expand that a bit, do *everything* the right way. Wear your uniform the right way. Always hustle. Play for your teammates. Sixteen hundred wins later and it's safe to say the system works.

I have many fond memories of playing catch with my father in the front yard. Almost any father will tell you that the first time you play catch with a son or daughter is a transcendental experience. It's the passing of the torch, circle of life kind of stuff. My son is a pretty good baseball player with a really sweet swing and a great glove. He's a solid pitcher too. More than anything I hope he can learn some of the lessons about teamwork, effort, and doing things the right way as he plays the game. However, people like Coach Schultz don't come around all that often.

Jack and I were watching the World Series a couple of weeks ago and Edgar Renteria hit the game winning homerun. There was a microphone in the dugout and you could almost feel the euphoria come through the TV screen. It was absolutely electric. He had just produced the game winning hit in his second World Series. I said to Jack, "I hope someday you'll get to experience what it's like to win a game for your team. The love you have in that dugout is just about the best feeling in the world." Because along with those great moments, there are times when you fail and let your team down. Those moments are important, too. You have to be willing to take your turn at bat and risk the pain of failing on the big stage. Facing that kind of pressure cannot be duplicated in a biology lab or a social studies lecture. That's why I learned more about life on a baseball field than in a classroom while I was in high school. All these years later and I still have so many fond memories of my time playing for Coach Schultz. I'd give anything for Jack to know what that feels like.

3. The laughter of children – There are certain things that always, but always, make me feel better. Pasta, sleep, and Diet Mt. Dew immediately come to mind but nothing can improve my mood as quickly as the sound of a child's laugh.

    There's a YouTube video that I like entitled "Hahaha." It's a short video of a child in a highchair laughing hysterically every time someone makes the sound, "bing." Apparently I'm not alone because the video has 146 million hits! There have been days where I've sought out the video when I'm in a crappy mood. After watching it, I always feel better.

    I often wondered if there is some genetic link that makes us all feel better at the sound of laughter. Could it be that laughter makes certain neurons fire in the pleasure center of our brains? Everyone likes to laugh. Why else would people dole out money to watch comedies on the big screen or go to comedy clubs?

Part of the reason a child's laughter is so intoxicating is that when kids laugh, they laugh with every ounce of their being. There's no polite chuckle. It's all or nothing. Children aren't afraid to just get lost in the moment. If they fall over laughing or poop themselves, so be it.

I think I'm drawn to childhood laughter because of my former job as a school psychologist. I spent my days tip-toeing through the minds of very damaged little people. My impressions of humanity are forever colored by those experiences. I need to remember that not every child will be exposed to the trauma of child abuse, parental divorce, and the types of loss that most of us were lucky enough to avoid until we were much older. I need to remember that children still find joy and light in the world.

4. The Iowa Hawkeyes – Cut me and I bleed black and gold. Actually that's not true. I stare down at the dialysis tubes three nights a week and there's no black or gold. It's all crimson red but I'm sure you get my point. My love for all things Hawkeye knows no bounds. But given the family I was born into, I never really had a choice. By the time I was old enough to have memories, my oldest brother, John, was attending Iowa earning a bachelor's degree before completing his degree in dentistry. A couple of years later, brother Jim, followed him to study medicine. Lyn was next in line and off to college she went to study nursing before emerging with a degree in journalism. My sister Lee Ann married her high school sweet heart, Doug, who was attending (you guessed it) Iowa to study pharmacy.

For some reason I never actually attended Iowa. I'm not exactly certain why. I think I was afraid it would be so awesome that I'd be overwhelmed. To me, Iowa City was like Mecca; a holy land to be visited on occasion but the thought of living there seemed impossible. I should also mention that the University of Northern Iowa offered me a suitcase full of money for a graduate assistantship. Still, I should have gone to Iowa at some point.

What I love most about Hawkeye athletics is that we're the eternal underdogs. The Hawkeyes never land the prize recruits. We never get the best athletes. Iowa takes the leftovers from the elite programs and then molds a great team with the kids that other schools don't want. And the Hawkeyes do it year after year with great coaching and a belief in "team first" which has become known to Hawkeye fans as "the Iowa way." The flashy four-star athletes don't come to Iowa and when they do they often leave because the Iowa way doesn't tolerate showboats. We like the humble native sons from Dubuque and Hiawatha who outwork the more gifted athletes. That's the Iowa way.

It's a kid like Dallas Clark who came to Iowa as a walk-on after receiving almost no interest from Division I schools. He started out as a linebacker, which is why he wears the unusual number for a tight end of 44. The coaching staff decided Clark may fit better as a tight end so they switched him after a short time at linebacker. The coaching staff was right because Dallas Clark was a phenomenal tight end at Iowa. After his junior year he won the Mackey Award which is given to the nation's most outstanding tight end. He left Iowa after only three years and was selected in the 1st round of the draft by the Indianapolis Colts. Dallas Clark went from walk-on, to starter, to All-American, to Mackey Award winner, to All-Pro…that's the Iowa way. Viktor Frankl, author of *Man's Search for Meaning*, said that people invent meaning for their lives. I think he was right. Looking forward to a big game has added spice to my life since I was a little boy and that love will continue until I no longer have breath in my body. Rather than being buried in some peaceful cemetery, I'd much rather have my ashes scattered in Kinnick Stadium in Iowa City, Iowa. Sacred ground. Go Hawks!

5. Dogs – My love for dogs has grown exponentially over the past decade. You see, I have a confession to make. For many years, I was a cat person. Please don't judge me too harshly. I have a good excuse. We started to acquire pets at a time in our lives when we were very

mobile. We could pack everything we owned in a small U-Haul and head out for destinations unknown. So it only made sense that our first three pets were cats. We didn't have kids yet so our cats were part of the family. Our male cat, Herb, passed away six years ago and we still talk about him all the time.

Cats have one huge advantage in that they are so much easier to take care of than dogs. You can leave cats for a few days and as long as they have food, water, and a litter box, they're good. They don't seem to have all that much affection for us humans anyway. At least they're not going to show it. But a dog has no issues about PDAs (public displays of affection) and that is what turned me into a dog person. There are so many things I love about dogs. I love the fact that dogs go absolutely bat shit when someone even says the word "walk." You could be watching a baseball game and say to the person sitting next to you, "I hope the pitcher doesn't walk this batter." That's enough for all the dogs within earshot to have an epileptic seizure brought on by the thought of getting to go outside and pee on everything.

I love the fact that male dogs will hump anything. Yes, I do mean anything. Our dog, Roscoe, has been fixed but even in his "ball-less" state, he constantly trying to get it on with our other dog, Myrna. I've seen dogs hump couches, pillows, book bags, suitcases and just about anything else within their perimeter. My wife tells the story of her childhood dog, Chip, humping air. Dogs do exactly what's on their mind and there's a tremendous freedom in that.

I love coming home from dialysis at 5:00 a.m. and who's waiting just inside the door with tails wagging? Not my wife and kids. Myrna and Roscoe are overjoyed that Daddy's home and now they can really stretch out a get some serious sleep. Actually I love coming home anytime and seeing their wagging tails in the front windows. I always know somebody's happy that I'm home. You can't buy that kind of loyalty.

6. Music – I can remember exactly when music became my master. I was in fifth grade and started listening to the radio when I went to bed. One night I heard the song "Takin' Care of Business" by Bachman-Turner Overdrive and something happened. I felt the hair on the back of my neck stand up. What was this rush I was feeling? I was hooked and all these years later music is just a huge a part of my life.

A few months later I asked (actually begged) my parents to buy me an electric guitar for my birthday. They assumed I'd mess around with it and give up but I was head over heels in love. I took lessons for about a year from a nun named Sister Sharon, who was as far removed from the stereotypical "mean nun" as you could get. She was teaching me "Down in the Valley" and I desperately wanted to rock. I asked her if she knew the chords to "Iron Man" one day and from the look on her face I knew my time with Sister Sharon was drawing to a close. I figured out that she couldn't teach me what I was aching to know so I struck out on my own with various books about music theory and improvisation.

What followed was the typical scenario of a music lover. I played in local high school bands with friends from my home town. In college, I had a band called "The Cause" and we were actually pretty good. I have a CD that we recorded and whenever I put it on I'm always pleasantly surprised that it doesn't stink. I had a plan to follow my muse all the way to Los Angeles which was the center of the music world at that time. I can also remember the exact moment I decided that a career in music was not going to be for me.

My band was playing at a venue called Matter's Ballroom which was one of our favorite places to perform. The place was absolutely packed with around 800-1000 kids. The Cause had a very positive message for kids. We were all about self-determination and following your dreams. We wanted nothing to do with the all-too-common image of drug-addled musicians who only worried about partying. In fact, we drank Diet Pepsi when we performed!

We were onstage playing the song "Born to Win" when I noticed these kids in the front row who had blood on their foreheads. They were so amped up from the music that they were slamming their heads together. They were headbanging in a literal sense. The one young man actually had white foamy material at the corners of his mouth. Yes, he was foaming at the mouth. I realized right then and there that these kids weren't getting the message. They had completely lost the ideas we were trying to convey. I had no interest in being another band that was indistinguishable from all the others. If The Cause couldn't be about something, if we couldn't be great, why bother? I decided what these kids really needed was not another guitar player. I could serve them better as a counselor.

I actually spent about ten years trying very hard to leave music behind. I didn't buy CDs or listen to music all that often. As I look back at that period and I realize what I was trying to do was grow up. It was a plan that was doomed to fail. Giving up music was like trying not to be interested in the Hawkeyes. As John Lee Hooker famously sang, "It's in him and it's got to come out of him." So I dove back into music with full force. I am now lucky enough to have a little home recording studio so I can create when the mood strikes me. Sadly, the mood has gone missing since I've been on dialysis. If I ever get healthy again, I'm definitely going to record some more music. I play guitar and listen to music all the time but I don't have the drive to write and record new music. Someday.

Of course there are lots of other things I will miss when I'm dead and buried. Some things are so obvious I decided to skip them. Suffice to say, the thought of being separated from my wife and kids is just about too much to bear. That's why I'm still fighting. I owe it to them. When I die, my problems will be over. My family will have to pick up the pieces in my absence. I am determined to make that a long time from now.

SOMEBODY DOWN
HERE LIKES ME

I'm not quite sure what to make of this but at this very moment there are several people who have volunteered to donate a kidney. Only one is a family member and none of them owe me a substantial amount of money. I just don't know what to make of it. Trust me, as Garth and Wayne say, "I'm not worthy! I'm not worthy!"

I've already told you about Curt Deckard. Out of the blue, he contacted me and offered me a kidney. Things were progressing nicely until his second set of labs revealed a problem. His blood work came back and placed him in the pre-diabetic range. I had never heard of the term so I did a little research and found that pre-diabetic means that a person's blood sugar level is higher than normal, but it's not yet increased enough to be classified as type 2 diabetes. The really scary part is that without intervention, pre-diabetes is likely to become type 2 diabetes in 10 years or less. If someone has pre-diabetes the long-term damage of diabetes, especially to the heart and circulatory system, may already be starting. So…shit.

At that point I immediately said, "Well, that's it. There is no way Curt can be a donor." As it turns out, the doctors at IU Hospitals did not share my pessimism. Pre-diabetes doesn't mean people *will* become diabetic, only that they *may* become diabetic in the future. The plan was to have Curt lose twenty pounds and see if the labs had improved. At this point, Curt has not yet reached the goal of that first twenty pounds. I've dieted a time or two in my life and I know the first weight you lose is the easiest. It gets increasingly difficult the closer you get to your target. Suffice to say if he's been trying for several months to lose the first twenty, the last twenty are going to be very difficult without a radical change of plans. I'm starting to wonder if Curt is going to be able to donate a kidney even if his pre-diabetic condition can be corrected with weight loss. I know he wants to but the people who run transplant programs have to keep the health and recovery of the donors as a priority. The last thing in the world I would want is for Curt to help me out and then have kidney difficulties of his own.

Around the time that Curt offered to donate a kidney, Dave Wiebke, an old college buddy called and asked about the process of being considered as a match. He had already been through the process of being considered as a bone marrow donor. Dave never said, "I want to donate a kidney to you," only that he wanted to be evaluated. So I gave Dave the phone number for the donor coordinator. A few days later he sent me an email saying that the donor coordinator told him that they don't start a new evaluation until they are finished with the one in progress. I remember thinking that was odd. If you have anyone who wanted to find out about living organ donation, why would you brush them off? Maybe he could donate to someone else.

Soon after the email from Dave, I found out that Curt was a match so I didn't give it much thought. As the months went by waiting for Curt to lose weight, I started to think more and more about Dave's email. Again, it just didn't make sense. There's such a need for organs. Finally I called my transplant coordinator and relayed the story to her. She immediately said, "That's not correct. We never turn away anyone who wants to be evaluated. Let me find out what happened and get back to you." A couple of hours later Tina called back and said, "There was some type of miscommunication between different staff members here. Someone will be calling your friend today."

I quickly contacted Dave and told him to expect a call. I also told him that if he was no longer interested that it was totally cool. He's got a wife and two kids also so this was not something he should go into without carefully considering everything involved. They called Dave later that night and he explained that he definitely wanted to continue the process. A kit for collecting blood samples was sent the next day and Dave scheduled an appointment to have the twelve viles filled. Twelve viles! Those transplant people are serious.

He texted me a couple of days later saying that he had been to get the blood drawn and there was nothing left to do but wait. My wife tried to find the words to express her gratitude. Dave was gracious and texted that he "hoped our blood wouldn't fight." I texted back, "We both know my blood could kick your blood's ass." So now we wait. I really do think my blood would win in a fight but let's hope it doesn't come to that.

Meanwhile, another friend from back in elementary school emailed that he wanted to be evaluated to see if he could donate. Kirk is one of those friends that it may be five years between contacts but when we do get together it's like we've been hanging out every day. There are no awkward pauses. I guess those are the kinds of friends who have known each other for a very long time. I talked to Kirk also about the potential risks. He said, "If I can't help out a friend I've known for almost forty years then what the hell am I doing on this earth?" Kirk is a retired military man so my stories of complications after surgery didn't worry him in the slightest. He said, "I've survived two wars so I'm not too worried about it." He makes a good point.

I just don't know what to make of all this. What the hell? I always thought that down deep I was kind of a self-absorbed prick. Apparently I'm awesome and had no idea. But trust me, I know I'm not worthy. I *know* I'm not worthy. My wife was telling a friend of hers about this and the friend said, "That just goes to show the type of person your husband is." Truth is I am very, very lucky to have friends like this.

Update from Dave

One week after having his blood drawn, I received a call from Dave. He told me that he had just gotten off the phone with the coordinator of organ donation for IU Hospitals. She had informed him that we were not a match. Just as I suspected, my blood totally kicked his blood's ass. Dave said she really didn't get into too many details about antibodies and the specifics of why it didn't work. It doesn't really matter I guess.

Another trip down on the emotional rollercoaster. I try not to think about things like this because it can be so devastating when things don't work out. Still, you hope against hope that maybe lightning could be caught in a bottle for a second time.

I could hear in Dave's voice how disappointed he was. He *really* wanted to be a donor which, again, just amazes me. You'd think there would be a sense of relief that he wouldn't have to go through all the hassle involved but there was none of that. If there was, he was hiding it pretty well.

I found myself in the all-too-common position of trying to cheer him up which I did by teasing him about how bad my Packers had recently throttled his Vikings. I can really be a jerk sometimes but at least talking about football and pictures of Brett Favre's penis changed the mood a little bit. Dave said, "I know how optimistic your wife was. Give her a hug for me." Damn, I have great friends.

Dave texted me this morning with a link about a paired kidney donation chain that he saw on the news in Minneapolis. He said, "This is too weird to be a coincidence." Since he can't be a donor for me, he wants to look into being a donor for someone else so that perhaps there would be a match for me somewhere out there. I have no idea how this works but I know it's a process that is being used more and more these days. It makes sense. You can't help your friend directly but by donating to a stranger, your friend is eligible to receive a kidney from someone who is a match. Some of these chains get very long and quite complicated. The story from Minneapolis is of a five kidney chain. So out of the disappointment of not being a match, five people get a new lease on life. How cool is that? So I have no idea where this is headed but we're going to finding out. It could be an interesting ride.

So Many Donors, Such Lousy Luck

Things are out of control. There are now *four* additional people who have stepped up to the plate to be evaluated to see if they are a potential match. Perhaps I've found the perfect level of vulnerability at work. I really don't know. I also think these chapters, which I am publishing as a blog, have been getting quite a bit of attention. People know the story and they feel a sense of responsibility because, through my blogs, they are aware how miserable I am.

Brenda

A few nights ago I was in dialysis and it was late. I guess I should say it was "later" because when your treatment starts at 10 p.m. it's always late. I checked my Facebook page and I had a message from a friend from my hometown, Brenda Burke Kochevar. I grew up in a town of about 1000 people so we really got to know each other going through school together. I have known Brenda since I was in kindergarten. Brenda wrote that she had been thinking about it and had decided that she wanted to be a donor. She'd been reading the blogs and decided that she wanted to be evaluated. Brenda is a nurse so I was relieved knowing she understands the risks and had obviously thought long and hard about this before deciding. I immediately had a feeling, "This is the one." I have no idea why that thought jumped into my brain but it did. I was floating through the rest of dialysis that night. I got home at 5 a.m. and had to resist the urge to wake up Polly and tell her the news.

My elation was short lived. I received an email the very next day that Brenda had mild hypertension that was well controlled but since she was on blood pressure medication, she could not be a donor. What's interesting about this is that she had talked to one of the transplant doctors she works with and he had told her that mild hypertension is not an exclusionary clause for the doctors at the Mayo Clinic. So mild hypertension is okay for the docs at Mayo, but not for the ones at IU? So…shit. I believe the clinical term for this is "covering your ass." I fully understand that hypertension is the leading cause of kidney failure but you can't tell me that the docs at IU know more about this than the docs at Mayo. So my next task will be to find out if I have insurance coverage at Mayo Clinic. If so, maybe a little trip to Rochester is in order. That's close to my home town so it would be kind of cool to get some bodywork down at Mayo.

Polly

My wife and I had talked about the possibility of her donating. I remember saying, "Not a chance. One of us needs to live." Well, after spending nine months on dialysis, my "ideals" have gone completely into the toilet so when Polly said, "I'm going to call the number and see if I could donate," I said, "I think that's a great idea." No time for heroics now. I need a damn kidney and I will swallow my ideals when necessary. It's amazing what misery and the fear of death will do to you.

Polly is probably one of the healthiest people I've ever known. She's never been sick besides an occasional cold. The only time she's been in the hospital is when she was delivering our children. But in the past six months or so, the stress of my situation has started to get the better of her. She used to have really low blood pressure and but she developed slightly high blood pressure and was prescribed a diuretic for it. Well, taking a water pill is enough to get your ass thrown off the list of being a potential donor. I said to Polly, "Tell them let me donate to my husband, make him well, and watch what happens to my blood pressure." I know her BP is stress related due to my situation. So, Polly is not an option and maybe that's for the best.

Missy

My niece, Missy, had expressed interest in being a donor but like I've said several times already, I don't know what people mean by, "I'd like to help you out." Missy and I talked about it a few times and I assumed that was the end of it. Now she is all fired up and wants to be evaluated. She also asked her father an interesting question, "Why aren't people in the family stepping up to help Uncle Jer?" All he could say was, "I don't know." And it may seem odd to people but I had never really thought about it until Missy brought it up. Why isn't my family stepping forward to be considered because I have a large family?

This disease, whatever it is, is definitely genetically transmitted. All three of us "Wilde Boys" have it. No one knows exactly who it will strike next or if it will continue but there's a very good chance that it will. I believe my family is hesitant to be considered for a donation because they may be afflicted with this disease later or perhaps they will need to donate a kidney to a member of their immediate family like a brother or sister. My brother Jim and I were talking on the phone a few days ago and he brought up the same question, "Why aren't more family members being evaluated?" I proposed my theory to him and he said, "Well, that may be true but we should tackle this as a family. If someone in the family donates and then there is a problem later on, then the next person in the family steps up and donates." He made an interesting point about our brother-in-law's family. Doug's sister Jody has kidney disease and when she became ill her mother donated a kidney to her. Jody had that kidney for several years and when it eventually failed, her brother Danny donated another kidney to her. I know that's how Jim wishes our family would react. I don't blame anyone for wanting to keep their original parts. That is double true when kidney disease runs in the family.

Maybe they are hesitant because they know what a jerk I am! I'm just kidding. I have been given so much love and support from everyone in my family. I know they are with me on every step of this journey.

Pamela

Then late last week a colleague from work stopped by my office to say she had been thinking about it and were going to be evaluated. Pamela Whitt has had a whole bunch of health problems since she arrived on campus three years ago. When she told me I said, "But Pamela you've been through enough. You don't need to have any more surgeries. I'm not sure you'd be eligible with all you've been through."

She told me, "All of my problems have been skeletal. There's nothing wrong with my organs dear." (She liked to call me dear.) So Pamela is taking the plunge.

Carla

Our administrative assistant Carla Bowen stopped by my office to tell me she also had contacted the donor coordinator to ask about donating. They told her during the initial phone interview that she needed to lose 14 pound in order to be eligible. I have no doubt that Carla will lose that weight. I'm just…WOW! I just don't know what to say.

I do have an idea why people at work might be willing to consider donation. It's because they see me every day. They see that I've basically become a shell of a man. I know it hurts to watch someone you love suffer and there is no hiding my suffering from my co-workers. They know when I say, "I need a minute" and run off to my office that I'm about to have another itch attack. The people in my family are so far removed from me that they don't have to confront the "new me" on a daily basis. It's easier to forget when I'm not staring you in the face.

I've had plenty of time to reflect on things (eighteen hours a week to be exact) and lately I've been questioning why it so hard for me to accept that there are people who are trying to save my life. Once I strip away the layers of false humility the best answer probably comes from my upbringing.

I grew up the youngest of five kids in a lower middle class family. Older brothers and sisters often do an excellent job of keeping younger siblings humble. My brothers were sixteen and fourteen years older than me so when I was working on my multiplication tables, John and Jim were finishing their doctoral degrees. They set the bar pretty high and, of course, my parents were extremely proud of them. The seeds were sown for an inferiority complex. I'm sure that's part of my misgivings about receiving a gift that would mean another chance at life.

The other thing is the magnitude of the sacrifice. It's not like I'm asking someone to watch our dogs for the weekend or letting me borrow a power tool. I'm getting a *kidney* which is slightly more significant than loaning me a shop vac.

Intellectually I know this is a gift that is given, not earned. It's little bit like getting into heaven. None of us can earn our way through the pearly gates. We all fall short of the mark. It is through grace we are saved. I'm counting on grace in this world and the next.

I have no idea how this is all going to play out but it's been a transcendental experience to have so many people volunteer to undergo surgery for me. If I make it through this, I have a responsibility to be the kind of person they see in me. And in all honesty, I'm not sure if I can do that but I am hoping to get the chance to find out.

THE END OF MY ITCHING

Just when I thought there was no hope of every living a life that wasn't preoccupied with itching, a small miracle happened. I feel like Lazarus; like I've been reborn. There are times when words absolutely fail to capture the feelings I am having and this is one of those times.

I had been trying to get some relief from the itching for several months. At first I tried using over-the-counter medications like Benadryl which did not work at all. In fact, for some reason, taking two capsules of Benadryl made me very agitated and jumpy. One night my dialysis doctor was in the middle of making his 100-yard dash through the unit (he tries to get in, see all of the patients, and get back out in under 10 minutes) and one of the nurses said to him, "Mr. Wilde is having all kinds of trouble with itching." I would have never brought it up, but Lori mentioned it and he came over to my bed and said, "I'm going to prescribe something that will help you. This will make you a happy man," he said in a way that actually made me think he might be right.

"This is a drug called Cholestyramine and you will take four grams twice a day. You have to take it with food. The pharmacist will explain that to you," he said.

I was confused by strange feelings of hope. He spoke with such confidence and conviction. He also wanted me to check with my liver doctor to make sure that I could take Cholestyramine before he would prescribe it.

A few days later I had a large package of Cholestyramine and, according to the pharmacist, I had to eat this drug with applesauce. That's not a great starting point for a romance with a drug. Obviously this was a "nasty" drug because if a patient were to take it on an empty stomach, bad things would follow (most likely the "two Ps," pain and puking).

I poured the requisite 6 oz. of applesauce into a bowl and sprinkled the magic powder on top. I braced myself and dug into the now greenish tinged applesauce. Of course, it tasted like death and had a slight metallic aftertaste. I couldn't have cared less. It could have been a steaming pile of poo and I would have done my darndest to eat it. Twice a day I celebrated this little ritual and soon discovered that the best way to cope was to pile it into my mouth as quickly as possible. No need to savor this stuff. Just get through it as soon as possible.

After about a month of using Cholestyramine, my symptoms had actually worsened. Like a good patient, I gave it my best effort because I really, really wanted some relief. Eventually I realized that Cholestyramine was not the answer to my prayers. I decided to see my doctor and perhaps he could make a referral to a dermatologist. I saw my general practitioner and explained my symptoms of extreme itchiness coupled with excruciating pain when I perspired.

He said, "Jerry, I have no idea what this is. I've never even heard of anything like this, but that doesn't mean I'm not going to try and figure it out. I have a couple of friends who are dermatologists and I'll call them and see if they have some idea." I really appreciated Dr. Black's candor. He's a GP and can't possibly be an expert in every disorder known to mankind. Whatever this was certainly wasn't your everyday "winter itch". To make it official, I started to perspire and went ahead and had a full blown "going ape shit" itch attack right in his office. I even stripped off my shirt, shoes, and socks so I could scratch like a deranged monkey.

He prescribed an antihistamine called Fexofenidine. This seemed logical to me as antihistamines are the drug of choice for itching. He explained that he wasn't sure this was going to help but this was a good place to start. All of this made perfect sense to me. I like Dr. Black and I always believe he's going to do whatever he can to help me. The plan was to take this medication for a week and then call his nurse to report how it was going.

After one week I tried to contact his nurse by phone to tell her that I was getting no relief. But I was kept on hold for twenty minutes before I hung up and tried again. I couldn't even get to her voice mail so, disgusted, I gave up and said, "Screw it." I decided I was going to have to figure this out on my own.

I decided I was going to try using a sauna to sweat out the poison. I had no idea if this would help but twenty years ago I remember a time when I sweated my butt off and for the next several days my itching was better. So my wife went online and found a sauna in Richmond. There appears to be exactly one. I wasn't sure exactly where I was headed but, after a few failed attempts, I found the Richmond Athletic Club and paid my seven dollars to experience excruciating pain. I was hoping that the heat in the sauna would make the process quicker but, no luck. It was still incredibly painful until I got a heavy sweat going. They recommended not spending more than 30 minutes in the sauna so I did my time and exited into a freezing cold shower. The cold shower wasn't part of the therapeutic regiment. I just couldn't get any warm water to come out of the shower head.

I was hopeful that my itching would be at least somewhat improved but the next day when I had another bee sting/itch attack I knew that the sauna was not the answer. I came up with a new plan. I had been reading about the use of tanning beds in the treatment of pruritis, the medical term for itching. Before I could get into a tanning bed I knew I had to go climb on the treadmill, induce the itch attack, and *then* try to give myself skin cancer. There was no way I could have laid in that tanning bed without having an attack. I did my ten minutes in the cancer-giver and went home. I knew I would not get any relief after one treatment.

Then I had an epiphany. I have a brother who is a doctor. He's actually a really smart doctor and I'm fairly certain he loves me a whole bunch. Why not call Jim? It's hard to explain why I hadn't thought of this earlier. Well, actually I had thought of this earlier; months earlier in fact. I just hate to put him in the situation of having to be in the role of brother and doctor. For some reason I am hesitant to turn to him for medical advice because I feel like I shouldn't trouble him. It's stupid I know and I need to do some real soul searching to figure out why I feel that way. He always says, "It's no trouble. I'm happy to help." Heck, my family calls me when they have questions for a psychologist. Why am I reluctant to get advice from a world-class physician…for free no less?

So I explain the symptoms to my brother. He says he needs a day to do some research but he'll get back to me. A day later he calls and says, "What you need is a drug called Gabapentin. Take 100 mg. after each dialysis treatment." I call Dr. Black's office and politely tell him what I need. It wouldn't have surprised me in the least if Dr. Black had said, "Well, let your brother call in the prescription," as I don't think anyone likes to told what to do and that certainly includes doctors. But to his credit, he faxed in the order for Gabapentin. To be perfectly honest, I wasn't terribly optimistic when I took my first dose at 5 a.m.

I woke up three hours later and I was dizzy. Not falling down dizzy but dizzy like, "Whoa! Who's spinning the world?" I managed to stagger into the shower and I started to notice something. I wasn't itching. I felt pretty "out of it" but I didn't care. I wasn't itching. Holy Mother of God, I wasn't itching!

Once I determined I was okay to drive, I went to work as I had to teach a class that day. It's hard to describe what I mean by feeling "out of it." It was a little bit like having an out of body experience. It was like I was in a movie watching myself. I wasn't particularly bothered by how I felt but I was glad I was only giving a test that day and didn't have to teach. One of my students asked me, "Are you okay, Dr. Wilde?"

I said, "Yes, I just started taking an anti-seizure medication so I feel very strange but I'm not itchy. You know how I'm always scratching myself up here? Today nothing itches. I feel absolutely great," and then we got on with the business of taking a final exam.

The added bonus to not being itchy is that I can sleep. The past few nights I've actually slept like a normal person. I haven't done that in a long time so I'm in the process of catching up on missed sleep for the past nine months. While I am aware of the fact that this "cure" may be temporary, I am extremely grateful to have a break from this torture. I am fully aware of the fact that it is "always something" with dialysis patients. The other shoe will drop eventually but right now I am enjoy the peace of mind my brother has allowed me to experience.

BY THE TIME I GET TO ARIZONA

There was a story in the news recently about transplantation in Arizona. I almost missed it myself and as you might suspect, I have more than a passing interest in transplantation stories. The good folks at CNN have started to report on this story and what I have learned sends a chill right through my bones.

Governor Jan Brewer and the Republican state legislature voted to stop financing certain transplant operations under the state's version of Medicaid. State officials said they recommended discontinuing some transplants only after assessing the success rates for previous patients. Among the discontinued procedures are lung transplants, liver transplants for hepatitis C patients, and some bone marrow and pancreas transplants, which altogether would save the state about $1.2 million a year. Critics have argued that the information provided about success rate of transplants was seriously flawed and in some cases, downright false. For example, the state said that 13 of 14 patients under the state's health system who received bone marrow transplants from nonrelatives over a two-year period died within six months. Outside specialists said the success rates were considerably higher, particularly for leukemia patients in their first remission. When I first read the "13 out of 14" data I *knew* it was wrong. I am not a doctor. I am certainly not an expert in transplantation but I *knew* there was no way that was accurate. How could the state officials in Arizona not sense that something was wrong? These are the men and women we elect to lead us, right?

There are about 100 people in Arizona who have been handed a death sentence by Governor Brewer and the state legislature. That is not hyperbole on my part. This is a death sentence, plain and simple. Consider the case of Mark Price, father of six. Just before the October 1 deadline, Mark Price learned he needed a bone marrow transplant to treat the leukemia that was killing him. On the very day that the new rules went into effect, a donor was found by his doctors. But on October 1st, Mr. Price no longer qualified for coverage.

As family, friends, and doctors scrambled to save his life, an anonymous financial donor stepped forward and agreed to cover the costs for Mr. Price's surgery. Just when it appeared that Mark Price would get the new lease of life he'd been waiting for, he died before the operation could be done. Remember the "death panels" that Chuck Grassley and Sarah Palin warned us about? They are here. They are functioning in Arizona. The only difference is that they are being propped up by the same people who spew about the "sacredness of human life." The Republicans are the "right to life" crew, correct? There seems to be a serious disconnect here.

What word can be used to describe conservatives who give lip service to the "culture of life" and then pass a budget that actually denies life-saving treatment to people? Hypocrite doesn't quite cut it, does it? This issue plays out when the debate about abortion comes up too. Conservatives are vitally interested in having all children born but don't appear to be all that concerned what happens outside the womb. They seem to love the unborn but they're not so fond of the adults out walking amongst us. When you get past the rhetoric and examine conservative policies, phrases like "family friendly" and "pro-life" have a hollow ring to them. Sure, pro-life *sounds* great! Who the heck isn't pro-life? But pro-life should mean more than just anti-abortion. If people are pro-life then their support for a child shouldn't stop when the baby is born. With many conservative policies, it does. The sick and dying in Arizona are just the latest example.

Let's be clear about something. Arizona has the money. It's only 1.2 million dollars! In a state budget ($9 billion annually) that's a mere pittance. Governor Brewer and her Republican colleagues are consciously *choosing* to let these people die. There will be more Mark Prices. But what did Governor Brewer and the state legislature choose to fund? Well, for starters, they appropriated $1.25 million to build bridges for endangered squirrels over a mountain road so they don't become roadkill. The project is expected to save approximately five squirrels a year.

But perhaps there is hope. A man from Illinois, Steven Daglas, has created a website (www.arizona98.com) where he describes 26 ways to restore funding to this program. Some will jump to the conclusion that Steven Daglas is a liberal whose primary motivation is to embarrass Governor Brewer. In fact, Mr. Daglas is a Republican Party official from President Obama's district in Illinois but that doesn't matter. As Mr. Daglas says, "This isn't a Republican thing or a Democrat thing. It's a human thing." Mr. Daglas' is quick to point out that as a conservative, he only considered ideas that would not take funding away from anyone else. His 26 suggestions were developed after paging through the Arizona's 9 billion dollar budget, line by line, and finding ways to save the money. If a man from Illinois can find ways to restore the funding, why can't the Arizona legislature? I'm still hopeful that the Arizona 98 will receive the life-saving transplants they need. I don't believe in guardian angels in the traditional sense with wings flying around us keeping us safe from harm. But I do believe that people have the capacity for self-less acts of love such as the work performed by Steven Daglas. I'll take Mr. Daglas in my corner any day, wings or no wings.

SO THIS IS CHRISTMAS

Things are in full Christmas prep mode here. The dialysis center got into the spirit of the giving, too. When I went in for my treatment there was a gift bag on my bed. Everyone likes to get presents so I dug into mine. The first thing I found was a carrying case for medicine that was shaped like a large pill... cute. There were several pieces of hard candy too which was a nice idea. Lots of dialysis patients carry sacks of candy with them during treatment to help with dry mouth. There was also a poem written to fit into the classic "Twas the Night Before Christmas." I have to be honest; I never made it past, "Twas the night before Christmas and all through the unit." That was it for me. I absolutely hate it when people who aren't on dialysis try to do something cute about dialysis. For some reason that really pisses me off. I always feel like they don't have that right. It may be a little bit like our African-American brothers and sisters feel about the "N" word. As patients, we can joke about dialysis but we don't like it when the doctors or nurses do the same. I saw a cartoon in the unit with a picture of Santa in a dialysis chair. Santa had a look of frustration on his face. The nurse in the cartoon was saying, "Three hours is three hours no matter what day it is." The date on the calendar in the background was December 24th. I absolutely hate that shit. Every time I look at it I am compelled to get a pen and write, "Ha-fucking-ha." Dialysis isn't a joke. We go through living hell to get through six hours on the machine and there's nothing funny about that.

Let's get back to the gift bag for a minute. Do you know what the "big present" was? They gave us giant water bottles. There are very few people on the planet who have to worry about consuming *too* much water. We are they. So they gave us water bottles. Was it supposed to be a joke? Why in the hell would they give water bottles to dialysis patients? That's like giving an alcoholic a fifth of vodka. "Remember to watch your fluid intake. Here's a half-gallon water bottle! Merry Freakin' Christmas!"

This Christmas week is a tough one on everybody here, nurses and patients alike. Nobody wants to spend Christmas day on dialysis and certainly no one wants to take care of a bunch of sick people on the 25th. Everyone wants a day off to celebrate Christmas. So they juggle most of the patients around so everyone can make December 25th a dialysis-free day. This leads to lots of confusion and frustration. Our schedules are shuffled around and routines are interrupted which means many dialysis patients are in a bad mood. We don't like coming in at different times. We don't like different beds. We *hate* coming to the dialysis center and the one thing that can make it worse is when our routines are interrupted. Or so it would seem. But the *real* reason we're in bad moods has nothing to do with being in a different bed or having to come into dialysis at an unusual time.

We're in pissy moods because Christmas is just another reminder of what has been taken from us. It's a reminder of what we gave up when we lost our ability to survive without dialysis. Most of you have the one gift we crave more than anything in the world…health. It's the most precious gift anyone can have.

Lots of people will be gathered together with family for Christmas. Not me. I'll be stuck here in Richmond missing my family in Iowa. Logistically, I cannot make it to and from Iowa given my need for dialysis. It would be almost impossible to drive ten hours to my father's home and then make it back to treatment Sunday night. Plus, twenty hours in the car sounds like a great way to celebrate the birth of Jesus.

As you sit down to a huge Christmas feast, remember we can't have mashed potatoes. And ham has lots of preservatives that we should avoid. Turkey is fine. A little wine is okay but not too much. Is that cheese on the green beans? Damn. Now we can't have the green beans. Oh well. We can always feast on the banana bread. Whoops! That banana bread might stop our hearts. Gotta stay away from the potassium. It's a killer. That's okay. Maybe we'll just stick with the turkey.

It doesn't matter if it's Christmas, Easter, or even if Jesus H. Christ himself decides to join us for dinner, we *never* get to forget our affliction. It is our burden to bear. And during special times of the year like Christmas, the burden gets just a little heavier. We'd give anything just to have a day off from this life. We live lives of thirst, both literally and metaphorically, but mainly literally. I'd kill to be able to drink my weight in Diet Mt. Dew. Someday.

So as my family digs into our presents, I already know the one thing I desperately want won't be under the tree. The present that can never be wrapped up with a bow is my freedom, my peace of mind, and my health. I'd sit on Santa's knee and beg if I thought it would help. I won't be doing that because Santa's not real. Plus I've always been a little freaked out by the Santas in the malls.

So take a minute this Christmas season and be thankful. Be very, very thankful you're not one of us down at the dialysis center. I hope you get everything your heart desires. Take a minute and say a prayer for those of us who know going in that we won't be receiving what we want. Not now anyway.

IT'S ALWAYS SOMETHING (MORE FUN WITH FISTULAS)

By now you've probably figured out that a dialysis patient's health is a pretty sketchy deal. Tenuous, unpredictable, and ever changing captures it quite nicely. We can be fine one day and then everything goes to hell in a hand basket a few days later. Either your labs are all screwed up or you're itchy as heck or your catheter is infected or your blood pressure is through the roof (or basement). It never ends. We're constantly waiting for the next bit of bad news.

As you may have surmised from the title of the chapter, the latest drama is my fistula. For those of you who don't remember, a fistula is the surgically altered vein used as the point of access during dialysis. In laymen's terms, it's where they stick the gigantic needles. A fistula is created by fusing a vein with an artery so the vein has increased blood flow. This also causes the vein to increase in size giving the appearance that you are smuggling a garden hose under your skin. Seriously, it looks like you're illegally smuggling cable TV into your chest. My fistula took two surgeries before it was functional. After the surgery is performed it takes about six weeks for the thing to heal and "mature" as the doctors say. These things are a necessary evil and they act like an expensive sports car: always acting up and constantly needing attention.

I've already had plenty of issues with this fistula. Like I said, it took the docs two cracks at it before it worked. For months I had to mess around with a catheter in my chest. Several doctors told me that patients get better dialysis when they are using a fistula as opposed to a catheter. They were absolutely right. After they started using my fistula I felt better almost immediately. But now there seems to be a problem. My fistula is big…too big. One of the nurses, Lori, had been concerned that it was ballooning out under my arm pit. She would say, "That doesn't look right." After a couple of weeks they decided I should get an ultrasound. Great…the last time I had one of those things they found a tumor. What were they going to find this time? I hope it's my missing set of car keys.

When I scheduled the appointment the nurse on the phone said, "Make sure your lower extremities are clean." This confused me. Why would my lower extremities have to be clean for an ultrasound on my arm? I started wondering, "Is this one of those things where they run a wire from your crotch up through your main artery? Oh crap. I bet that hurts like hell." I asked her, "I'm confused. Why do my lower extremities have to be clean?" In typical administrative speak she said, "I don't know. I'll transfer you to someone who can answer your question." I was on hold long enough to imagine all sorts of grizzly things they might want to do to my lower extremities. Of course, my lower extremity is also the general location of my penis. Anxiety rising. Why are they trying to damage my penis? My penis is sick enough already.

At that point a lady answered and said, "Yes, can I help you?

I explained I did not understand why I needed to clean my lower extremities.

She said, "It just helps the ultrasound device pass over the skin easier."

I said, "But the problem is my fistula in my bicep."

"Oh," she said. "Well then just make sure your arm is clean." My penis breathed a huge sigh of relief.

The ultrasound itself was non-eventful. A few days later I was down getting my blood cleaned at dialysis and one of the nurses, Heather, gave me a piece of paper. I asked, "What's this?"

She said, "Oh, your ultrasound results were abnormal so they've scheduled a procedure."

"What kind of procedure?" I asked.

"It's called a fistulagram. They make a small incision on your arm and run a wire up there to clean it out. They might have to do a kind of angioplasty too," she explained.

I had heard of the dreaded fistulagram before but not by that name. Dialysis patients refer to it as "where-they-run-a-freakin-wire-up-your-vein-and-it-hurts-like-a-mother-o-gram." Damn. It's always something. Seriously, I have talked to a few dialysis patients who have had this procedure and all of them mentioned it was painful.

I've now got a few days to convince myself that all those other patients were just pussies and that I am able to withstand anything they can throw at me. So far it's not working too well. It'll be okay because at the end of the day all I have to do is transform myself into an inanimate piece of meat and hold still on the table while they give my arm the Roto-Rooter treatment. Piece of cake. After all, how painful could it be to have a wire run up your vein from your arm through your fistula? Sounds like a walk in the park to me.

But I do have a question. Who decides which procedures get mild sedation and which get the "here's a bullet to bite on" treatment? There must be some type of protocol but I have no idea what it is. All I know is that on New Year's Eve day I'll get the business and hope like hell they can fix whatever it is that's wrong with my fistula. If this thing fails, it's not a tragedy but it would involve more surgery that I don't want. The docs have used up my left arm so they'll have to start hacking away at my "good arm." This would mean they'd have to put another catheter into my chest until the new fistula heals. It would also mean that for the rest of my life they'd have to use my leg to take my blood pressure. I had my BP taken through my leg one time and it was very strange. It actually hurt quite a bit. I thought something was wrong with the machine but it was just that I wasn't used to the anaconda treatment on my leg. I'll let you know how this turns out.

Post-Op Report

I've had a day to recover from the fistulaogram. In short, it went fine. By that I mean it didn't hurt too much. From a medical standpoint, it was unsuccessful. So what else is new?

They got me into the room where they were going to conduct the procedure and it was very cold. That was excellent because it decreased the likelihood that I'd have an itch attack while they were plumbing my pipes. The doctor performing the procedure was very nice. She explained exactly what they were going to do and throughout the procedure asked me if I was in any pain.

The procedure took over an hour because first they had to put dye in my fistula to find the parts that were too narrow. While the dye was in there they took a bunch of pretty pictures. Then they angioplastied the heck out of my fistula to try to open it up. Sadly, it didn't work. After all that time, they managed to increase the width of my fistula by one millimeter. One freakin' millimeter. They did their best but sometimes there is not much they can do to increase the width in the narrowed portions of the fistula.

So after it was all said and done, they started to clean me up. They had a large drape over my face the entire time so I wouldn't see what they were doing. That was a good idea because I probably would have freaked out had I been watching. I knew I was bleeding quite a bit because, while I was numb at the point of entry, I could feel the blood running down the sides of my arm the entire time. When the drapes were finally removed I was stunned at the amount of blood I had lost. Holy Shit! I thought someone had snuck in and gutted a deer in the operating room while they were working on me. No wonder I felt kind of weak after the procedure. I'd better have some red meat for lunch.

Let me say for the record that I'm very, very fond of my blood. We've had some great times together. I want to keep it with me at all times. In the end, all I got out of this was a large bill for my insurance company and a killer bruise on my bicep. At least they were nice and let me listen to classic rock on the radio while they Roto-Rootered me. That was a bonus. No Christian rock this time!

COME WALK
WITH ME IN HELL

As I wake each morning, a question automatically forms in my mind: "Is this a dialysis day?" If it is, there is a certain dark resolution that sets in that colors the hours until I leave for my treatment. I know what is waiting for me. Thoughts of needles, blood, and cleansing pop into my mind periodically throughout the day.

The second question is, "How bad will the itching be this morning?" Within a couple of minutes of waking my hands and feet start to itch. Remember back a few pages when I was glowing about my itching problem being under control? Well, you can forget that because it is back with a vengeance. I'm not sure why. Maybe my body has become accustomed to the medication. I did finally make an appointment with a dermatologist but that is not for three months so I've got a lot of pain and scratching to get through. Lately I've been drawing blood during these sessions and actually breaking finger nails.

The itching comes on slowly in my hands and feet. Will it last five, ten, or fifteen minutes? Will it spread all over my body or be contained to my hands, feet, legs, and arms? This is my routine. You know how some people get up, go to the bathroom, and brush their teeth? I scratch myself bloody.

The use of the word scratching would lead you to believe my skin is itchy when that is not really true. As I've explained before, my skin feels like I am being stung by bees. I scratch and that does something to stimulate the particular nerve that is acting up. The problem is that there are literally dozens, if not hundreds, of nerves firing simultaneously all over my body. It appears as though I am playing an unusual game of "whack-a-mole" with my skin. I am losing the game. I need more arms. After a particularly long and painful session my hands are cramping up from exhaustion.

Yesterday was particularly difficult day in terms of itching. I was awakened at 4 a.m. by an "itch attack." It spread all over my body and would not dissipate. I went into work at 8:30 a.m. and damn it, I had another itch attack in my office. I closed the door, took off my clothes except my pants, and displayed an impressive array of scratching techniques.

I endured a long meeting with Marilyn, my boss, about accreditation. I can honestly say without any hesitation that I'd rather have my teeth cleaned than plan for accreditations visits. Marilyn makes it tolerable because she is so committed to making sure we "make it." It's a tremendous amount of time and energy. The rest of the day was inconsequential. I went for a "fake bake" session to see if that might provide some relief from the itching. It did not.

Fast forward to the evening: I leave for dialysis at 9:30 p.m. but I have to start getting ready approximately 45 minutes prior. That is the time required for the lidocaine gel to numb my arm. The gel usually works quite well. It doesn't take away all the pain of the needle but it helps.

Applying the gel is a family affair. After I carefully dab on the right amount, my daughter helps me get the Glad Cling-Wrap into place around my left bicep. Anna has become a suitable "pinch hitter" when my wife is gone. Anna is happy to lend a hand because she loves me so much and wants to do anything she can do to help me. The cling-wrap keeps the gel from getting all over my clothes and also from drying out. I am very appreciative of this magical goo. The last time I was on dialysis there was no numbing gel. Needles were just jammed into my forearm. Hurt like hell, too.

I start to gather my "dialysis equipment" which consists of my iPod, keys, license, benedryl, soda, and a book. Tonight I am fried and know that I will not be in the mood to do any reading so the book stays home. I watch some TV with my kids while I keep an eye on the clock. Finally it is time we exchange hugs. The kids will be on their own tonight which rarely happens. Polly is in Nebraska with her father. We found out that he has cancer in his colon and liver. Mel is 83 and living on his own in Nebraska with only a niece in the area. Right now, more than anything, he needs his family around him which is a challenge since we live three states away. My kids are 16 and 13 so they are able to spend a few hours without adults around but I hate the idea of them being alone. If something were to happen, it would take me at least 30 minutes to arrive home. This is only the second time we've had to leave them over night and I hope it is the last. When you add my father-in-law's illness to the mix, to say that this has been a shitty year would be an understatement.

Knowing they will be alone tonight we go over the emergency plans once again. "If there's any kind of problem, what are you going to do?

"Call you," Anna says.

"If I can't get here quickly enough, who are you going to call?" I drill them.

"Eloise and Bob," Anna repeats like she is reciting a line from a play she has rehearsed many times.

"If it's a real emergency, what are you going to do?" I ask.

"Call 911 and then call you," she replies.

I have good kids and they are very responsible. Still, I hate the idea of them being home alone overnight. Our two dogs would disembowel anyone trying to get into the house. At least I think they would. They may just want to receive "pets." I'm never quite sure. Their bark is probably way worse than their bite.

The hugs are a little bit longer and a little tighter tonight. Jack actually gives me two hugs. There are times when there is an unspoken, yet unmistakable, fear in his eyes. I know what he is thinking. "What if my Dad dies?" My boy is a worrier. He always has been and this health problem certainly hasn't helped. I am conflicted about the messages I send to him. I try to reassure him that I will make it through this but, the truth is, I may not. What will be the effect on him if I've promised him I'll survive and, in the end, I don't? Can a child ever believe anyone again after that kind of breach of trust? These are hard questions and despite all my training and experience as a child psychologist, I am not certain what to do. When it comes to your own kids, all that training and experience seems to fly right out the window. Here I am not Dr. Wilde. Here I am Dad.

In the end, he needs to believe with every fiber of his being that his father will be okay. So that is what I tell him and quickly regale him with stories of all the things we're going to do when I get healthy. I love those moments. I love the look in his eye when he is believing- when he is absolutely trusting- that his father will be just fine and we'll be doing all the silly shit that fathers and sons do together again. And, yes, a lot of it will involve urination. I have promised him we'll go into the backyard and pee on every tree on our property. We're going to send a message to every dog in our neighborhood that the big dogs are back.

I double and triple check that I have all my dialysis equipment and head out the door. The drive takes 15 minutes depending on how lucky I am with the traffic lights. Tonight the roads are a little slick from the snow we've had so I am careful. What would I do if I slipped off the road? I do not want to find out so I am extra careful. I like to pull into the parking lot by 9:45 p.m. because I want to be on the machine by 10 p.m. That way I can be getting off the machine at 4 a.m. When I get to the last traffic light before I turn into the parking lot, I can feel my spirits drop. Shit. There it is. The Fresenius Dialysis Center used to be a grocery store. The dialysis center takes up the left half of the building and an eye doctor's office the right. I find my normal parking spot (third slot in the last row facing out so I can head straight out after treatment...no backing up for me!) and briefly scan the parking lot for the stray tomcat that used to be around. I haven't seen him in months but still, it would be great if he'd show up one more time. Maybe someone adopted him. I pick up my back scratcher from the passenger seat and head into the building.

As I hit the entry way I often mumble the phrase, "Come walk with me in hell," because this is my own private nightmare. I have this bad dream three times a week. Very few things frighten me anymore because I've seen this dark side of life. I have a feeling that this is going to be a bad night. The last few have been that way. Dialysis treatments are never good. Some are easier to get through than others. No matter what, I've got to get through another treatment.

So while the rest of the country is enjoying themselves at home or out with friends, I am about to be connected to a machine for six hours in order to remain alive. I walk through two sets of automatic doors that always remain open far too long once you've passed through them. They are set for wheelchairs, not ambulatory people. The TV in the lobby is always on although at night, there is never anyone watching. There is a coat hanger on the door keeping it open which allows those of us scheduled for nocturnal treatments to walk right into the dialysis area. The rest of the patients who have day treatments have to wait to be called. Suckers! I hang my coat up and immediately notice that Chad, the 20-year-old who sits in the first row of chairs, is not in his normal location. When someone is absent my heart skips a beat. This could be good or it could be bad. My first thought is always, "transplant?" which is odd because it is much more likely to be hospitalization or some other problem. Still, my first thought is always that maybe they've received the ultimate gift. As it turns out Chad was in the next row of chairs where Sam usually sits. Big Sam was out of town on business. Damn. No celebrating here tonight.

I hang my coat up and begin the process of weighing in and taking my temperature. The ear thermometers require you to put a little plastic ear condom on them to stop the spread of ear diseases. I look into the case and one of the ear condoms is loose in the package so I put it on the thermometer and jab it into my ear. After the beep I take it out of my ear and the ear condom actually stays in my ear which is the first time that had happened. I approach the scale with fear and loathing. My weight has been up lately mainly because I haven't been running as much. I do not sweat anymore so why run? I mount the scale and try all my tricks to keep the number from being too high. Do not make direct eye contact with the scale. It doesn't like that and punishes such displays of hubris with big numbers. Holding your breath usually helps so I did that too. Read 'em and weep time. 76.8 kilograms! In less than two days I've gained almost 10 pounds of fluid. That is too much for me and my fears of a bad treatment have been kicked up a notch. Damn. I'm drinking too much soda.

I walk to my bed and start unloading my dialysis equipment before I climb in for the longest six hours in the world. I say "hi" to all the usual cast of characters. It is quiet on the unit. I looked over to Henry's bed to see if he was restrained. Remember Henry? He's the guy who pulled out one of his needles and sprayed blood all over the place a couple of months ago. Two nights ago we had a repeat performance. There was not as much blood this time and they did not have to call an ambulance. I was wondering if his hands would be restrained tonight. They were not.

It looks like Trey will be putting me on the machine tonight. That is good. He is good with the needles and once told me he loves drawing blood. This is the perfect job for him. I climb into the bed and wait to see if my hands and feet will itch. They do but not too badly. Trey collects all the necessary needles, gauze, and other materials before starting. He puts on the tourniquet and my fistula becomes huge. A blind man could get a needle in that thing. Trey wipes down my arm to get all the lidocaine gel off before sterilizing it. He feels around for a few seconds looking for just the right spot before closing in for the poke. I always watch because I hate waiting for the pain. I want to see everything so I know exactly what's happening. He told me once I'm one of the only ones who watch the needles being inserted. It's surprising how much force it takes to get the needles into the vein. It's easy to break the skin but to puncture the wall of the vein is another story. The nurses try to deliver the right amount of pressure without pushing too hard. They are trying to avoid putting the needle all the way through the vein once the wall gives way. It's same kind of situation when you are trying to open a bag of chips. You want to pull just hard enough to get it open without shredding the bag once it opens. Alright…one needle in, one more to go.

As Trey is feeling around for the second entry point, I realize I can feel his fingers on my fistula. Damn. I must not have gotten enough lidocaine gel on the upper part of my arm. This one is going to hurt. He picks out the spot and, bang, it goes in easily this time. Not only did it slide in easily, it didn't hurt a bit. Awesome. Needles are in. That is good.

He's playing around with the tubing and my phone rings. This rarely happens because it's 10 p.m. and most of my friends are asleep by that time. I'm afraid it is Anna and there is a problem. I check the number and it's my wife.

Polly says, "Hi, honey. I know you'll be leaving for dialysis soon so I just wanted to call before you took off."

"Honey, I'm at dialysis. I just had my needles put in."

"What do you mean? It's 9:30, isn't it?" she asks.

"No, it 10 o'clock," I say.

"Are you sure?" she asks because between the two of us, she is usually right. We both know this so we often defer to her judgment.

"I'm looking at three different clocks so, yeah, I'm pretty sure," I say.

As it turns out the battery on her watch is failing. She apologizes about five times but it is nice to hear her voice. There is no news about her father.

Trey injects some saline solution through one of my needles and asks, "Does that feel okay?" It does so he connects everything and I'm ready to go. He starts the dialysis machine and I watch my blood flow down the tube into the filter which quickly turns crimson. A short while later the blood is through the machine and headed back into my arm. Everything is working as it should. Now it's just a matter of keeping things that way.

I had decided on the way over I was going to watch a concert DVD from a band I like called Lamb of God. I own the DVD but someone also posted it on YouTube. I call up the first segment of the DVD and the band is playing "Laid to Rest." For this moment I am able to forget I am in a dialysis facility. Instead I focus on the fact that I could be doing this at home. The only difference is the location.

I've watched this DVD here in treatment a few times so the bloom is off this rose. I watch the first hour and stop. That's the best part anyway. What to do now? I'll check Facebook. Nothing earth shattering there. I try to pick a fight with one of my Facebook friends. I'm not sure if I know this person but I think she's from my hometown. Actually I'm not sure. She posted a link that slammed Nancy Pelosi and the Democratic Party for running up the deficit. I post under the link, "Damn democrats…what we need is a few wars to stimulate the economy." I'm sort of hoping I can bait someone into posting comments back and forth. I've got five more hours to kill so I'm willing to do just about anything to pass the time. No luck. I check back throughout my treatment but not a lot of people are trolling Facebook during the middle of the night.

The next few hours pass sloooowly. I am comfortable except for my arm. The needles actually hurt a little bit tonight which is rare. I keep checking to see if everything looks okay at the access point and it does. No swelling. No leaking. Just a little bit of pain.

Around 2:30 a.m. I decide I should sit up for awhile. My ass is totally asleep and I need to change positions in this bed. As I expected, I start to get another "bee sting" episode. It begins with my hands and feet as always but quickly spreads all over my body. I'm in a mild state of agony now as my body is covered with invisible bees doing their worst. One of the nurses stops over and asks if I'm okay. "Just the itches again. I'll be okay." The nurse who is usually in charge, Lori, is out sick tonight. I miss her during times like this because she occasionally comes over, puts on gloves, and scratches my back. This allows me to concentrate on the rest of my body. For some reason when she comes to help me I think of the Bible passage, "*For I was hungry and you gave Me food; I was thirsty and you gave Me drink; I was a stranger and you took Me in; I was naked and you clothed Me; I was sick and you visited Me; I was in prison and you came to Me.*" With Lori it would be, "*For I was itchy, and you scratched me.*" It's always a little more of a problem when I have one of these attacks while I'm on the machine because I essentially have only one hand for scratching. The pain is bearable this time and after a few minutes I am able to lie back and just scratch my feet and hands. I can manage if it's just my hands and feet. I am hoping that this latest episode will keep me from having a "bee attack" while I'm being taken off the machine. I rarely have these episodes back-to-back so this was a calculated move on my part. Why am I the lucky one? No one else here has to deal with these episodes.

The last couple of hours take an eternity but finally I am within fifteen minutes of getting off the machine. I decide to sit up to see if the bees will attack again. I slowly sit up and wait. My feet itch a little but my strategy appears to be working. The bees are sleeping. Shhhh!

The needles come out and my blood pressure is good. The last few treatments have left me weak and dizzy because of dehydration. Lori decided that my new dry weight should be 72.5 kilo and that appears to be just about right. I get my needles removed and hold my "wounds" for five minutes before taking a peak. You have to be careful because the blood flow out of a fistula is significant. It's basically an artery dressed up like a vein. I have stopped bleeding so I tell Heather I'm ready to be wrapped up in bandages. She comes over and tapes up my arm which still hurts for some reason but it doesn't matter now because I am DONE. It is hard to describe the joy of being done with a six hour treatment. Yes, I know I will be back in two days but that is long time from this moment. Now I get to go home and that sounds great to me.

I take my temperature again and climb back on the scale. I have lost ten pounds in six hours. How's that for a diet? I say my goodbyes to everyone and slowly walk toward the door. There is a shuffle that dialysis patients all share after a treatment. It's hard to describe precisely but it's a little slower than normal. Feet shift along the floor rather than being lifted up. We've just had all our blood taken out of our body and cleaned. We're not quite feeling …normal.

I head out and see Sue in the lobby. I always hope she is gone for two reasons. 1) She's been here with the rest of us for a long time. She wants to go home and get some rest, and 2) I am so worn out that sometimes it's hard to find the strength to engage in thirty seconds of small talk. We talk about our plans for the weekend. Her daughter is her pride and joy and she will be with Sue this weekend.

Another bonus awaits me in the parking lot. My car windows have not frosted over. Right now, at this place in time, life is good. For two whole days there will be no doctors, no nurses, and no needles in my life. Plus, I don't have to scrape the car windows at 4:30 a.m. I am grateful for small blessings. I drive home being able to see clearly for the first time in weeks.

Normally I make an illegal right-on-red turn on my way home. Just as I'm about to break the law I spy a police car a block away and waiting in the dark. My luck is holding out tonight so I wait for the light to turn and slowly head home. As I pull into the garage I am greeted by the cat that has moved into our garage. She loves to stretch out on the hood of the car after I get home and soak in the heat. I am too tired to pet her tonight. She rubs her lips on the antennae hard. I think that antennae must owe her money or something. There is only one thing on my mind…food. I am famished after dialysis and tonight I have leftover macaroni waiting in the fridge. I walk in the door, greet my dog Roscoe, and head directly to the fridge. I toss the container into the microwave, hit 60 seconds, and drop off all my dialysis equipment. Each night I have a little race with the microwave. I try to have all my equipment stored before the microwave bell rings. As usual, I lose the race but the prize for second place is a steaming pile of noodles. I'll get you next time, microwave!

I slam down the noodles so fast that there are almost sparks coming of my spoon. I barely bother to chew them. It is a little past 5 a.m. now, bedtime. I tip toe upstairs and quietly check on the kids. Jack always sleeps almost completely wrapped up in a blanket. Only his face is exposed so even though he is quickly becoming a man, he looks like an angelic little child curled up in his bed. Down the hall I check on Anna. She is also asleep so I breathe a small sigh of relief. I have made it through another treatment and things are okay at home. I climb into bed with our dog, Myrna. Another day down…one day closer to a transplant. Goodnight world. A few hours later I will awaken and ask the question, "Is this a dialysis day?" On this morning, the answer is a resounding, "No."

GOD NEVER GIVES YOU MORE THAN YOU CAN HANDLE

There are certain phrases that just get under my skin (but "get under my skin" is not one of them). The title of this chapter is at the top of the list of those phrases. Before I start ranting and raving about it, let me start with a few other phrases I really dislike. Feel free to add your own at the end of the chapter. I'll leave some space.

Hate the Sin, Love the Sinner – I don't care for this one because it's so judgmental. We are *all* sinners, right? So when people say "Hate the Sin, Love the Sinner," essentially they are calling everyone a sinner. How is calling someone a "sinner" helpful? I know I'm a sinner. I don't need reminding. At least this one has good intentions—to remind people that we all fall short. I just don't like what the phrase implies. It makes me *want* to sin even more.

It is what it is – Not a big fan of this one either. It is what it is. What else could *it* be? It doesn't move the conversation forward at all. Plus, this phrase can fit into any discussion at any point so it's sort of useless, isn't it?

"I just got into law school."

"Well, it is what it is."

"I have a ripping roaring case of jock itch."

"Well, it is what it is."

"I can't find my car keys."

"Well, it is what it is."

Does anyone need that? You could just make up another completely useless phrase and it would work just as well.

"I just got into law school."

"Well, it's important to get enough fiber."

"I have a ripping roaring case of jock itch."

"Well, it's important to get enough fiber."

"I can't find my car keys."

"Well, it's important to get enough fiber."

Actually, I prefer *"Well, it's important to get enough fiber"* because at least people would stop and think for a second, "What was that? Did he say something about fiber?" At least you're providing good advice. Fiber *is* important.

God Never Gives You More Than You Can Handle - I'm not sure exactly when this started to bug me. It's probably because people throw it around so often. This phrase is what people call a "truism" but is it really true?

So when my mother developed lung cancer and had to have surgery to remove the tumor, was that more than she could handle? Nope. She was a tough old gal. Mom survived. Then after her lungs were clear of cancer but it spread to her brain, was that more than she could handle? Well, maybe because it spread all throughout her brain until she didn't even recognize her own family. Perhaps we need to define "handle." When she died a slow, agonizing death from brain cancer, did God give her more than she could handle? To me it would appear that death from brain cancer was more than my Mom could handle because it killed her. Death would appear to be the textbook example of "not handling it."

But God always has an escape clause. He allowed cancer to destroy my Mother but He took her to heaven so He's got eternity on his side. So, by default, He can *never* give you anything you can't handle. Even if it stone cold kills your ass, you can handle it. To my mind this is bullshit, circular logic but lots of mindless people go around mumbling *"Well, God never gives you more than you can handle"* and feel comforted. I have a better phrase. *"Remember, the death rate is still 100% so, screw it, nothing matters."* I can see the t-shirts now.

Okay, time for a chill pill. Maybe I need an attitude adjustment. Maybe my trials and tribulations are an opportunity to grow as a person. Maybe this situation is a "blessing in disguise" and will teach me valuable lessons about life. Hey, that's certainly true. I've had experiences through these illnesses that I could have never imaged otherwise. These challenges have had a profound effect on the person I am today. But, to be perfectly honest, I feel like I've already paid that bill. I've been through all this twenty years ago and anyone who has danced with death the way I have never forgets, or if they do, they are a certifiable asshole (or maybe just a bit crazy). I completely understand how precious life is. It seems like this latest episode is just suffering without the life lesson. Maybe I need to look harder. I could do without it, quite frankly, but I realize I'm not the one driving this bus. Maybe nobody is at the wheel right now. I just have one question for God: What lesson do I have to learn?

Is the lesson:

- **Preciousness of life?** Got it. Watching sick and dying people three days a week pounds that one into your brain.

- **Treat every man, woman, and child with respect and dignity?** I try so hard at this. I know I fail sometimes but it's not for a lack of trying. This is so very important to me.

- **Live each day as if it's your last?** I do my best. I don't waste time (other than Facebook.) Those of us living on machines have a much greater appreciation for squeezing the fun out of life whenever we can.

- **Importance of fiber?** (Refer to the first part of this chapter.)

- **Trust in the Lord?** Hold on! What was that one? Houston, we may have a problem. I can say unequivocally that I do not have complete trust in the Lord. I don't have complete trust in anyone or anything. That's not my nature. So is that it? That's the lesson? I have to trust with all my heart that things will work out the way God intends? That's going be a tough one.

I'm not the trusting sort by nature. What the hell? Nothing else seems to be working. Sure, why not? What have I got to lose? But if that's not it, could you send me a clue? I'm running out of ideas down here.

NO SWEAT

I'm not exactly sure what is going on but apparently I've lost the ability to sweat. I'm not sure exactly when this happened but for about the past month or so I've noticed that when I go for a run on the treadmill I barely sweat. Actually that's not entirely true. I sweat under my arms and in my lower abdominal area but nowhere else.

At first I thought, "Man, I'm really turning into a lazy bastard. I need to run harder." So, I cranked it up a notch. No sweat. Next I thought, "Maybe if I wear extra clothes that will get the juices flowing," so I put on three layers of clothes. No sweat. My next thought was that maybe my pores are totally backed up and what I need is a thorough cleansing. I had been to the local sauna a few weeks ago and sweated like a pig. So I headed back over to the sauna and hunkered down for what I thought surely would be a sweat-fest. Again, no sweat. I sat in that heat for 25 minutes and my arms, legs, and back were bone dry. I finally said, "Screw this. I'm getting out of here" and walked out of the sauna. I felt my stomach and, what do you know, it was moist. "Hey, I'm sweating," I said to myself. And then it hit me…I'm not sweating. The moisture was *condensation*! My skin's temperature was approximately 194 degrees compared to the locker room's 72. I was "sweating" the way a cool drink does in the summer. What the hell! I had practically baked myself and still couldn't sweat.

Not sweating can be a problematic for a few reasons. The first of which is obvious; sweating is what people do when they get hot. It's how they cool down. I've known people who had some type of heat stroke and do not sweat. My mother's face used to get very red when she got overheated and that was the sign that we need to get her out of the heat. I really hope I don't have to deal with this the rest of my life.

I used to run almost every day as a means of managing my itching but also as a way to sweat off excess fluid. That's not an option at this time so I have to be careful how much I drink. I've been heading into dialysis as much as 10-12 pounds heavier between treatments. That's too much for me and it's making the treatments difficult. I feel nauseous and am on the verge of cramping when they have to take that much weight off. Plus, I'm gaining weight (real weight…not fluid) which would seem to be a good thing after having lost 40 pounds following the surgery. Gaining weight while you are on dialysis is not good because determining what your "dry weight" should be is a guessing game. The only way to figure out patients are gaining weight is when they get sick and cramp up at the end of the treatment. You'd think there would be a better way but, if there is, I'm not aware of it.

The last thirty minutes of my most recent treatment were awful. I was on the verge of cramping the whole time. I yawned twice and each time got a little cramp in my throat. How weird is that? When I told the nurses I was starting to cramp they took my blood pressure. It came back at 90/45. So they gave me some saline and took my BP again. Same reading. I asked for some water and guzzled down a big glass. I felt a little better but my BP was still very low. More saline…sit around and try to make the room stop spinning…check BP…still way too low…more saline…sit around and wait…check BP…you get the picture. They won't let you leave until your BP is above 100. I finally rang that bell forty minutes after they started to take me off the machine.

I'm really hoping that this problem is simply another issue related to my extreme lack of kidneys. In the summer, I live outdoors. I'd hate to have to start limiting that. Well, there's no need to worry about it until summer.

WHEN THE PAIN COMES

By now I am sure you are getting tired of reading passages about my burning skin. I can't say I blame you but right now, it is my primary source of agony. I'm going to write about this one more time because I want to capture how these episodes impact not only me, but my entire family.

The pain comes each and every day. It is like the freakin' sun rising in the east. Count on it. Sometimes I am relatively lucky and I wake up to a massive attack. After enduring fifteen minutes of agony, I am through with the pain for the rest of the day. That is the best possible scenario. More often I have several small attacks until the "big one" comes later.

When the pain comes, I feel a sense of panic. Once the burning sensation reaches a certain intensity in my hands and feet, I know it is going to spread like a swarm of bees all over my body. It's inevitable. Once I feel it on my lower back, I know the next fifteen minutes of my life are going to be the worst pain I have ever experienced.

This morning I was at the computer checking my email before going to church. Not more than 45 minutes earlier I had an "episode" but it only involved my hands and feet. Sometimes these episodes will buy me some time before the full episode takes place. Not today. My hands and feet start to burn and—boom—it hits. I start pulling off clothing as I headed for the family room. I say to my son Jack, "I need help," and he knows exactly what he needs to do. His job is to scratch my back during this attack. I try to take care of all the other itches on my body. Having someone available to rake my back helps considerably because then I can concentrate on hands, feet, arms, legs, head and abdomen.

The intensity of the burning starts to increase. Try as I might, I am unable to simply take this pain and I started to cry out. Looking back on it now, I am surprised by the vocalizations I make when I am in this state of agony. At first I repeated, "Oh God," over and over again but I am not praying. For months I would pray, "Please God help me," during an attack but He wasn't listening. For some reason, "Oh God" is still the phrase that comes out.

After a few minutes I start to cry, "Come on, come on, come on." I try to think, "I can take it. I can handle this pain." After several more minutes I have no choice but to accept the fact that this pain is overwhelming and I feel even more desperate. I am looking for any sign that the burning pain is starting to wane. There are a couple of moments when I believe the worst is over and that the pain is subsiding. Then I reach the horrible realization that round two is starting. My vocalizations give way to mere cries of pain. I no longer attempt to use words. I am in full onset panic mode now. The phrase, "My God, My God…why have You forsaken me?" runs through my mind.

That is when I see it. I see the looks on my children's faces. It is a mixture of sadness that their father is being momentarily conquered by this pain but also looks of extreme unease. It's like a horrible car accident on the side of the road and they have no choice to look at the carnage. They look at me, their father, their protector, their hero, and see a broken, pitiful man. They see their father at his absolute lowest point.

My wife now takes over back scratching duties. I groan a "thank you" to Jack who quickly exits the room. Polly knows this routine. We go through it every day. She knows how to keep the neurons firing in the skin on my back so I can scratch where it is needed most.

I start to become exhausted. My hands are cramping from ten minutes of constant use. I am breathing heavily from the exertion it takes to scratch with this level of frenzy. Still, there is no sign of this episode abating. I start to get pissed. Pissed at God, pissed at my broken body, pissed at the millions of people who will never experience this level of agony, pissed at those same people for still complaining about silly shit, pissed at myself because I cannot "man up" and take this quietly. I am embarrassed by my cries of pain. In my mind, I am trying to convince the rest of me to remain silent but my mind is losing that fight. It's like my body is calling out on its own accord.

And then, after ten minutes of violent scratching, I notice a small reduction in the percentage of my body that is affected. My hands and feet feel as if they are on fire but there are parts of my legs that are burning with a lower intensity. I don't need to scratch them as frequently. This is a good sign. A few more minutes and this attack will be over. I consciously attempt to regain control over my voice and this time, I win. I whisper the refrain, "Okay, okay, okay" and my wife asks, "Is it getting better?" "Yes," I say.

I can slow my breathing now. I survey myself and look for blood. Both feet are bleeding from the opening of old wounds. My leg is also bleeding but not too badly. I will not need bandages to stop this bleeding.

Throughout the attack I keep asking, "What time is it?" because I know we have to leave for church. Anna and Jack are singing in the choir today. Polly keeps saying, "Don't worry. We've got time" and we do. The attack surrenders with a full ten minutes to spare before we have to leave. Now, I must redress myself as, during the attack, I got rid of all clothing except for my underwear.

I apologize profusely to my children for them having to see this event. I often have these attacks when no one is home or I am at work so they are spared. They shouldn't have to see their father like this. Anna and Jack reassure me that it's fine but I know better. When I was their age I couldn't even imagine my father in this state. The idea of my father being overcome by anything simply would not compute. He was a rock. Today at age ninety is *still* a rock. He reminds me that he could kick my ass if he needed to. He is probably right. As a child, my father's vigor gave me a sense of tranquility and confidence because no matter what, I knew my Dad would take care of me. He was, and still is, my hero. In my practice as a psychologist I saw thousands of kids whose fathers were anything but heroes and I felt grateful all over again for having a phenomenal dad. I am a far cry from the father figure he was and I wonder how that will impact my children later in life. I am not blaming myself because I know my broken body is not my fault but still, why can't my kids have the kind of father I had?

After the attack has been handled, my mood picks up considerably. A few minutes after the attack I tell my wife, "I am in a good headspace now." She looks shocked so I try to explain.

"It's because I've had this attack which means I shouldn't have another one for a few hours at least," I explain. "Also, I think being in so much pain helps the body release endorphins. I almost have a runner's high right now."

We pile into the car and head off the church. In the church parking lot Polly says, "The last thing I want to do is worship God right now. I feel more like going to a bar and having a drink."

I understand. She's pissed at God, too. I say, "If God's given me this terrible body, why would I worship him?" But people go to church for all kinds of reasons and some of them have little to do with God. I am afraid that perhaps my faith has been shaken so badly I will never fully recover.

We head into church and find our familiar spot in the balcony. I am in an almost joyful mood because I've had my attack and now I won't have to worry when I'm going to have it today. I have paid that bill…or so I think. About a half an hour into the service I realize I am starting to have another attack. I tell Polly I need to leave and slip out as inconspicuously as possible and head down to the bathroom. You know the routine by now. I strip to the waste and get down with the scratching. I am pleasantly surprised that this attack is more of an aftershock than a full blown earthquake. After putting my shirt back on I leave the bathroom and hear the rest of the sermon. Fingers crossed that this is the last one of the day.

I do not know why I have been given this lot in life. Is there a reason? Maybe, maybe not. Either way, that does nothing to change my present reality. Right now all I can do is pray for the strength to handle it with as much dignity as possible. These attacks aren't going away anytime soon.

AN ETHICAL DILEMMA

By now you should know Curt, the former student who has volunteered to donate a kidney and basically save my life. He's been diligently trying to lose the weight necessary to meet the guidelines to be a donor. Forty pounds is a heck of a lot of weight for anyone to lose. It's been about seven months since that glorious day when he showed up at my house to tell me in person that we're a match. While seven months may not seem like a long time, it's an eternity to a dialysis patient. It may sound like a cliché but it's a struggle to just make it through each day. So I think it's obvious why I have such an intense interest in young Mr. Deckard's weight. I'm not being nosy. I just want to live.

It's been difficult to get a straight answer from him regarding his progress towards the goal. In fact, I've asked him several times, "How close are you to the goal?" or "How much weight have you lost?" and he simply will not give me a direct answer. It's never, "I've lost fourteen pounds." It's always a little more cryptic. A few days ago he emailed to say, "I only need to lose seven more pounds to have my interviews with the surgeons." I'm not clear what that means exactly. Does that mean when he losses seven more pounds it will be a total of twenty pounds he's lost?

I am extremely grateful for Curt's incredibly selfless act. However, if I am being completely honest, there have been times when I was not sure if he would ever make his goal. Perhaps he'll get there but I'll no longer need a kidney because I'll be dead. So I have pursued multiple means of finding a match. My college buddy, Dave, wanted to be a donor but we were not a match. Dave was not deterred. He wanted to explore paired donation where he would donate his kidney to an anonymous dialysis patient as long as I would also get a kidney. Well, some time has passed and Dave's calls were coming less frequently. I emailed to ask if he was still interested. He's still interested but his wife is not. Can you blame her? What does she get out of this? An incapacitated husband. I've got nothing to offer other than the "contact high" of being incredibly proud of her husband and that only goes so far.

My high school buddy Kirk was interested in donating but several years ago he had a period of time when he was on blood pressure medicine. The folks at IU hospitals asked him to have his BP checked over a period of time and report the results back to them. Unfortunately, Kirk didn't make the grade. He called me at my office the other day so I knew he had important news. We made some small talk for awhile and then the phone line went silent. His voice was cracking with emotion as he said, "I'm not going to be able to get through this." I interrupted and said, "Bro, let me finish the sentence, 'I got tested and I'm not a match.'"

He explained, "No, I can't even get tested," and went on to explain that his blood pressure was too high. He was absolutely torn up that he couldn't help me. I was absolutely amazed he was taking it that hard.

Which brings us to another high school friend, Brenda, who would like to be considered to be a donor. She was told by the donor coordinator at IU Hospitals that she could not be a donor because she has also has a history of mildly elevated blood pressure even though it is well controlled through medication. She suggested that I find out if I have insurance coverage at Mayo Clinic, which I do. I talked to the transplant people at Mayo Clinic and they told me I would need to be in Rochester for about one month if I had the transplant there. So I had my blood drawn and sent via Fed Ex to the Mayo Clinic to determine if we are a match.

Here is my ethical dilemma. Do I owe it to Curt to keep him abreast of all of these other possible donors? What do you think? I can't decide.

On the one hand, I can feel my body breaking down. This being kept alive by machines isn't nearly as much fun as it sounds. I need to do whatever I can to survive and survival looks a lot like a transplanted kidney. On the other hand, holy shit, he's working to lose weight to save my miserable life. Doesn't he deserve to know every relevant bit of information? I can be such a selfish prick. But on the other hand, I need to know how he's doing with his weight loss too. I'm not being nosy. That information has a huge impact on my life. He's not exactly being forthcoming with me or I'm too obtuse to understand. Then again, lots of people don't like discussing their dieting successes and failures. Maybe he's tight lipped because he *knows* this is life and death stuff and he doesn't want to let me down.

See what I mean? This is classic ethical dilemma stuff. In the end I think it's safe to say that survival wins out. Yes, dear reader, I want to *live* and I'm doing what I think will give me the best chance of surviving. I am not telling Curt for the very simple reason that I'm afraid if he's aware that I'm pursuing other options he might slack off on his dieting. In the back of his mind he would be aware that someone else might be able to donate so he could relax a bit on his weight loss plan. But what I can't decide is whether or not that makes me an asshole. I do have a habit of expecting the worst out of people. That's not a personality trait I am particularly proud of but at least I'm consistent. I always assume people will take the short cut, have an excuse, or simply do the wrong thing.

I guess I can take the chicken shit way out and see what the lab work from Mayo Clinic says. It could be that Brenda's not a match. C'mon Curt. Seven pounds. What exactly *does* that mean?

THE END IS NEAR

The title of this chapter isn't referring to my demise. It's not the end of me, just the end of the book. This story could go on for months or even years and it's just going to be more of the same. Itching, needles, infections, thirst, cramping, buckets of blood, and an intense longing for the one thing that is beyond my reach... a normal life. It's just too damn sad and nobody would want to read a 300 page memoir about me.

My goal has been to give a glimpse into the life of a dialysis patient. Unless you've been there yourself or lived with someone on dialysis, there's no way to understand what it's like. It's not all that it's cracked up to be. But, as my father says, "It beats the alternative." Some days I'm not so sure but then I've had a good stretch on dialysis and I feel hopeful again.

I hope it's been a good story. If I've done my job, you've laughed a little and been moved by the struggles I've faced. I hope you've taken some time to reflect on the fact that *nothing* is more important than your health. And if you happen to have diabetes and/or high blood pressure, *please take care of yourself.* You don't want to become another name on the list. There's always room at a dialysis center near you. If it's overcrowded, they'll make room.

I must confess I had one other motive. I have always hoped that perhaps I could inspire some of you to consider donating an organ to someone in need. You know how I keep returning to the question, "Is there a reason for all this suffering?" Maybe that's why I'm driven to tell this story. In the middle of this very difficult time, I'm supposed to transcend my particular circumstances and think of the welfare of others. Would that make this all worthwhile? Who knows but if anyone decided to donate a kidney because of this book, I would strip off my shirt, beat on my chest, and give the Tarzan call. The willingness to help others doesn't have to be limited to a friend or family member. There are thousands of strangers waiting and their pain is just as real as a brother, sister, aunt, or cousin. If you are curious or have questions, please check out the website Donate Life America http://www. donatelife.net. Approximately half the states in the union have their own chapter of Donate Life so Google it to find the one in your area.

Another great resource is the website for the National Kidney Foundation http://www.kidney.org. There's a tremendous amount of information on just about anything and everything that pertains to kidney disease, dialysis, or transplantation.

Now, I must also admit that I feel somewhat bad for leaving you hanging. Seems like there should be one more chapter in this book, doesn't it? "But what happens in the end? Does he get a kidney, return to health, get discovered by a major league scout, and become the oldest rookie in the world to lead the Minnesota Twins to an improbable World Series title?" Well, it was a conscious decision on my part to end the book without the Hollywood ending. You know, good triumphs over evil, the guy gets the girl of his dreams, and I get a kidney and return to urinating like a mad fool. This story could go on for a long, long time. Remember what I said about survival rates for dialysis patients? About 25% of us die each and every year. By the time you are reading this I could be gone, baby, gone…surfing with Elvis as they say. But I do have a solution if you want to see how this story turns out. If you're interested, give me a call (765-994-1120) or look me up on Facebook… I'm the Jerry Wilde with a beard. You can also email me at jwilde@indiana.edu. If I'm alive, I'll get back to you. I promise. If the message gets bounced back to you it means one of two things: I'm dead or I found a much better job! It'll probably the former as I'm tenured and I have no intention of going through that again.

Okay, now the end really is here. Thank you for buying the book. I'd like to add that a portion of the profits will be donated to the National Kidney

Foundation. See, you're already helping and you didn't even know it. I'd like to close with the words of one of my favorite authors, Albert Camus.

In the midst of winter,

I finally learned

That there was in me

An invincible summer.

Best wishes and good health.

ABOUT THE AUTHOR

J erry Wilde is a professor of educational psychology for Indiana University East. Prior to this academic appointment, he worked as a psychologist where he counseled children who had emotional, behavioral, and learning difficulties. He is best known for his popular book *Hot Stuff to Help Kids Chill Out* which is designed to help readers learn to manage their anger. He and his wife, Polly, live in Richmond, Indiana with their children, Anna and Jack.

A documentary movie (*18 Hours*) about Jerry Wilde's story is being completed as this book went to press. *18 Hours* was directed by Dr. James Barbre III, a colleague from Indiana University East. Please search under the film's title at websites such as www.vimeo.com and www.youtube.com to watch portions of *18 Hours*.

BUY A SHARE OF THE FUTURE IN YOUR COMMUNITY

These certificates make great holiday, graduation and birthday gifts that can be personalized with the recipient's name. The cost of one S.H.A.R.E. or one square foot is $54.17. The personalized certificate is suitable for framing and will state the number of shares purchased and the amount of each share, as well as the recipient's name. The home that you participate in "building" will last for many years and will continue to grow in value.

Here is a sample SHARE certificate:

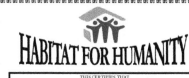

THIS CERTIFIES THAT

YOUR NAME HERE

HAS INVESTED IN A HOME FOR A DESERVING FAMILY

1985-2010

TWENTY-FIVE YEARS OF BUILDING FUTURES
IN OUR COMMUNITY ONE HOME AT A TIME

1200 SQUARE FOOT HOUSE @ $65,000 = $54.17 PER SQUARE FOOT
This certificate represents a tax deductible donation. It has no cash value.

YES, I WOULD LIKE TO HELP!

*I support the work that Habitat for Humanity does and I want to be part of the excitement! As a donor, I will receive periodic updates on your construction activities but, more importantly, I know my gift will help a family in our community realize the dream of homeownership. **I would like to SHARE in your efforts against substandard housing in my community!*** *(Please print below)*

PLEASE SEND ME _____ SHARES at $54.17 EACH = $ $_____

In Honor Of: _____

Occasion: *(Circle One)*   *HOLIDAY   BIRTHDAY   ANNIVERSARY*

          OTHER: _____

Address of Recipient: _____

Gift From: _____ *Donor Address:* _____

Donor Email: _____

I AM ENCLOSING A CHECK FOR $ $_____ PAYABLE TO HABITAT FOR

HUMANITY <u>OR</u> PLEASE CHARGE MY VISA OR MASTERCARD *(CIRCLE ONE)*

Card Number _____ Expiration Date: _____

Name as it appears on Credit Card _____ Charge Amount $ _____

Signature _____

Billing Address _____

Telephone # Day _____ Eve _____

PLEASE NOTE: Your contribution is tax-deductible to the fullest extent allowed by law.
Habitat for Humanity • P.O. Box 1443 • Newport News, VA 23601 • 757-596-5553
www.HelpHabitatforHumanity.org

Printed in the USA
CPSIA information can be obtained
at www.ICGtesting.com
JSHW082207140824
68134JS00014B/480